Candida
Yeast

Angela Kilmartin
www.angela.kilmartin.dial.pipex.com

First published 1995 by
Bloomsbury Publishing plc.

ISBN 0-9542677-2-9

This edition written and published
Angela Kilmartin
www.angela.kilmartin.dial.pipex.com
Copyright 2003

Library of Congress cataloging in
publications data.

Design, typesetting and print:
Bay Port Press,645-D Marsat Court,
Chula Vista,
CA 91911
Tel: 619/429-0100

Distributed: New Century Press,
1055, Bay Boulevard, Suite-C.
Chula Vista,
CA 91911.
Tel: 619-476-7400
Orders: 800 -519-2465
sales@newcenturypress.com

ACKNOWLEDGEMENTS AND THANKS

I would like to thank the following for their help in the research and preparation of this book:

The British Society of Mercury-Free Dentistry; Drs Len and Helen McEwen; National Institute of Medical Herbalists; Wellcome Institute Library; Westminster Library; Central Books Ltd.; Fiona Ross; Jack Levenson for all his mercury wisdom and my life back; David Harvie-Austin my anti-mercury dentist for clearing the Candida and fifty more symptoms of mercury poisoning.

My thanks are due for this edition to Lyn Patterson whose friendship and contacts in America have made the project very simple. Also to Ron Fraga, Cindy Alvarez, Bruce Collin, Linda Carter and Myra Ackroyd for their technical help in design, print, publicity and distribution.

Angela Kilmartin

CONTENTS

ABOUT THE AUTHOR

Angela Kilmartin's three careers have ranged from fashion model to opera singer to health campaigner. Her professional singing career was cut short in her twenties as a direct result of recurrent attacks of cystitis and Candida. However, as her knowledge of self-help grew, she began to fight back against these two seemingly insurmountable problems that for years had been ruining her career and marriage. In 1971, Angela founded the first bladder charity, known as the U&I Club, and produced a bi-monthly magazine for thousands of members. Between 1972 and 1994, she researched and wrote six books on cystitis and many leaflets and articles, and made two films. She also counsels, appears regularly in the Press and gives lectures.

Candida/ yeast has been inextricably entwined with everything she has done and her first six books contain much work on it. After nine years bed-bound by fatigue more Candida and awful ill health the diagnosis of mercury poisoning and safe removal of mercury teeth fillings resulted in a total resolution of all problems.

The accent of Angela's work is on educating both patients and doctors about the vital roles of self-help and prevention used in conjunction with conventional medical knowledge. The lifestyles of individual sufferers hold clues helping both sufferer and doctor achieve a correct diagnosis, and she hopes that this book will go some way towards helping identify important clues that will limit or stop the suffering.

Angela Kilmartin has a daughter and son and lives in London. All current books, written and published by her include this one and 'The Patient's Encyclopaedia of Urinary Tract Infections, Sexual Cystitis and Interstitial Cystitis'. Both are available or orderable from all bookshops and from the web. More information on these subjects and mercury poisoning is available on:

Website: www.angela.kilmartin.dial.pipex.com

urinarytractinfectionkilmartin.com

candidayeastkilmartin.com

1 Times past and times present

It has never been possible, right from my earliest days as a writer on cystitis in 1972, to exclude mentions of Candida. I was the first health writer to incorporate it in specific chapters on vaginal causes of cystitis, and my knowledge of it has greatly increased over the years.

As with those books I have written on cystitis, my interest in Candida and yeast infections has also been borne primarily from suffering and a desire to 'wreak revenge'. It is important that you should know the extent, involvement and triumph over Candida that I have had; it may comfort you to know that I have experienced first hand all the frustration, discomfort, medical consultations, clinics, treatments, social and sexual implications that are involved. For me, writing a book is a means of communication with another sufferer as well as offering ways of dealing with the problem.

Where it all began

I cannot point to a specific episode, month or year when I first became aware of Candida. This is because doctors in the 1960's were not on the lookout for it, and it might even have been as late as the second of my five years as a recurrent and acute cystitis sufferer that my doctor bothered to take a vaginal swab. I didn't even know such a thing existed!

Of course, the 1960's saw a dramatic change in many social and health issues. With short hemlines came nylon tights. New oral contraceptives met the demands of sexually-free young women, increasing food and drink choice followed post-war austerity and new antibiotics arrived for all sorts of infections. It was a time of many advances, and I was a child of most of them. That any of these advances might be hazardous to health was unthinkable; everyone was, and continued to be for many years, completely unaware of the unwanted and even dangerous effects of these exciting new discoveries and changes.

Some years on, things are different. Women working in the media, particularly in magazines and newspapers, write on a large variety of health-related topics, and we should all be hugely grateful to them for providing us with help and education in matters which, medically, can still often confound many male doctors.

Against this medical and social background, my own life as a young woman in her early twenties in the mid 1960s was busy and happy. I was an only child, convent-educated, musical, often lonely from asthma and bronchitis, poorly travelled and eager to get into life's mainstream once I left school at the age of seventeen and a half.

I met my husband during five years in the fashion trade and we enjoyed a three year courtship and engagement. Like everyone else, we slept apart and lived at home with parents. Apart from my allergic rhinitis and past asthma, neither of us had any minor or major health problems. Occasional snatched sexual encounters were wonderful and absolutely trouble-free.

Life promised great happiness. We became inseparable as months of courtship and mutual interests grew. My musical talents as a pianist developed into an interest in singing. Local operatic and dramatic roles led to scholarships and awards at the Guildhall School of Music and Drama in London where I quickly began taking lead roles.

By twenty-four years old I was facing a delightful life ahead with marriage and highly promising operatic career. It should have been blissful. But August 6th 1966, my wedding day, proved to be the starting point of personal tragedy, of enormous suffering and the breaking of faith in God as well as doctors. The marriage was dashed and damaged from the moment we made our vows. I had not just married Paul, I had become espoused to a cause, though I did not know it at the time.

Honeymoon cystitis prevented the honeymoon in Tunisia from being our first sexual holiday. From day two, I became incontinent and screamed with pain when passing bloody urine. Fainting, feverish and frightened, I was eventually carried to a woman doctor who diagnosed cystitis and prohibited sex, swimming, sunbathing, spicy foods and alcohol. An oral urinary antiseptic was prescribed serving only to colour my leaking urine blue on the white marble floor. Daily penicillin injections into my buttocks were painful. It was and remains a truly terrible memory not just of itself but also of what it came to symbolize over seven years of similar attacks. About seventy eight attacks took place in those dreadful years wrecking my singing career, my sex life and nearly the marriage, too.

Then, as knowledge dawned slowly, both the severity and number of attacks decreased, until 1976 when I achieved total control with self-help.

Candida, also known as Thrush, wove in and out of this awful scenario, probably from the honeymoon itself, but almost certainly from the end of that year. Because cystitis and antibiotic medications were non-stop, other perineal symptoms were barely noticeable. Had I known of Candida, I daresay I would have distinguished its symptoms from the pain, twingeing, aching, dryness and inflammation with me night and day from the cystitis. But I didn't know of the existence of Candida at all.

Magazines and health articles in the 1960s did not mention such taboo topics. Women's health was not a concern, either to the media, to the doctors (other than pregnancy and childbirth) or to us patients. Doctors knew everything, nothing was questioned. Medical textbooks, much as now, concentrated on research and surgery and were of limited help either to doctors or patients when it came to common ailments. There were no leaflets on either cystitis or Candida and no advice from any source whatsoever. The five minutes (at the most) spent in a doctor's consulting room was not for the patient to ask questions, even if she had the nerve to do so; such time was spent at the doctor's whim, writing prescriptions and expounding theories.

I spent a very great deal of time in surgeries between 1966 and 1976 reaching out for help in hospitals and Harley Street consulting rooms as well but the story was the same, no matter how much money was involved.

'Try these new, stronger antibiotics.'

'Take one a day for six months.'

'Take one at night.'

'Take four a day and stop sex for six months.'

'The infection can't have cleared we'll repeat the antibiotics.'

Antibiotics only brought in some twenty years before, certainly saved my life and prevented acute scarring of the kidneys, but they didn't stop those dreadful attacks of cystitis from starting in the first place.

At some point in the second year, my doctor at the time listened with great sympathy to a list of my symptoms: twingeing, swollen perineum; feeling as though another cystitis attack was about to begin all the time; needing to go to the toilet more than usual; hot perineal skin; a smelly, stringy discharge on my pants which seeped through to my tights; unbearable sexual intercourse although this didn't happen on many occasions; and agonising, almost orgasmic itching.

'It sounds like thrush, undress and I'll examine you.'

'What's thrush?' I asked.

'It can occur from taking antibiotics, we see more and more of it these days - once upon a time it was practically unknown, except when someone was gravely ill and their body was no longer able to cope with infections or overgrowths of fungi. Ah, yes!

There it is. It's quite bad and the whole area is very inflamed. The swab I'm taking will prove it, but I'm reasonably certain. I'll insert a pessary while you're lying down so that the pessary will be high up on the cervix. You'll need to insert one yourself twice a day and wear a sanitary towel to absorb the liquids caused by the pessary melting. The best time to insert one is at night since it can stay in place for eight hours, but this looks bad-you'll need two for seven days.'

Again, as with the cystitis in the early days, I thought nothing more of it. It happened once in a blue moon, was soon put right with a course of treatment and probably wouldn't happen again. I was so naive!

Just writing this is emotional; a step back in time to a bottomless pit of private pain and anguish. That August in 1966 was the start of everything that was to follow in my involvement with cystitis and Candida; it was the start of my apprenticeship with them both - a necessary apprenticeship for all the campaigning, writing, lecturing, counselling and publicity for the self-help approach that is the key to resolving these problems. Only such an apprenticeship - followed by blinding rage - could possibly realise the intense changes and struggles that have followed.

These two non-stop problems brought my marriage to its knees, my singing career to a stop, caused great depression and mounting anger.

The pessaries slowly started working towards the end of the week, but I was far from comfortable. My whole pelvic area felt raw, hot, itchy and slimy from the combined discharges of thrush and pessaries and then another attack of cystitis began.

Sexual intercourse, even when attempted on better days, was miserable. We were so much in love and so wanted a full physical relationship. Night after night, the new king-size bed stayed silent and unused except for fitful sleep, sobbing or scratching. We put up a reasonable front to the world, but countless social events were marred or missed because I was too swollen, too drugged up, too frightened of leaving the vicinity of the bathroom or too tearful to attend.

I've lost count of the hours spent at surgeries or hospitals; the vaginal swabs and urine samples taken to laboratories or doctors; the desperate Saturday-night trips to the all-night pharmacy in Piccadilly Circus for prescriptions; the endless hours spent crying in the bathroom.

My brilliant career prospects evaporated as it became obvious that not only was my voice itself losing lustre from pain, discomfort and drugs, but vaginal itching, discharges, pain and incontinence would physically prevent me from appearing on stage. In 1967 it reached a point when, after several close shaves, I was refusing to sign performance contracts. I was very frightened of committing to work of any kind.

Various operations on my urethra and bladder were tried without the slightest success. Antibiotics, permanent vaginal yeast/thrush, horrible drippy pessaries and pads, oral anti-fungal pills like Nystan were part of my everyday existence.

In 1968, despite our limited sex life, I became pregnant. I stayed home having occasional singing lessons, practising, doing housework and felt that until this dreadful time ended, I might as well have babies and then, ever hopeful of a cure, would be well enough to resume my career. My daughter was born in May 1969 under such appalling medical conditions and care that it took five years for me to pluck up the courage to have a second child, and even then it was only because we didn't want her to be the solitary child in the entire family. My son was born in May 1974. The obstetrician delivering him has publicly apologized for causing an inverted uterus and nearly killing me. It was a year before I was able to have pain-free sexual intercourse as a result of this trauma and the four hands of two obstetricians fighting to save my life.

Ever hopeful of a cure for the cystitis and the thrush, these two ailments dominated our little family. I could never predict when I would be free of them. In fact, the thrush never left me at all for years, easing slightly during anti-fungal treatments but always raising its ugly head again a few days later.

Vaginal thrush and gut Candida (which caused terrible wind) ruined my sex life for long after the cystitis began abating in 1971, finally ceasing completely by 1976 due to self help. But right through to 1982, I scratched nightly until the blood ran, refused almost all sex, shoved pessaries up to the cervix, took oral treatment for weeks on end, cried buckets and watched as the marriage ran out of stuffing. Yeast/thrush didn't go properly until my mercury amalgam fillings were removed in 1995 following years of additional fillings as life went by. Unthinkable that the trusty dentist could be adding to my woes!

There was nothing to read on thrush until I first mentioned it in passing in Understanding Cystitis, published in 1973. No leaflet or media articles were to be found, and the first book dedicated to it published in Great Britain only came out in 1984. By 1979, I was writing huge chunks about it from my own experience and information that had been gathered. The biggest chunks of knowledge were incorporated into my new books on cystitis and updates of older ones.

Fortunately, I have now recovered. There was a nasty time during a five-year struggle with so-called Myalgic Encephalomyelitis (ME) which turned out to be mercury poisoning from the accumulation of many dental fillings and the addition of four gold caps which caused galvanism. Even more mercury leaches out in the presence of a noble metal, gold, with saliva as the conductor of the electrical currents that this process creates. Systemic Candida added to the near-deathly fatigue, but thankfully I knew by then how to keep it vaguely under control. I now see people for counselling on cystitis, Candida and mercury poisoning.

So, you see, very few people could be better qualified to write about it than me. The best campaigners always start from personal involvement and I count myself as just such a one.

On that fateful morning of August 6th, 1966 I had a husband and my opera. God had given me a splendid voice and a life-long mate. I felt happy and blessed.

By 1969 I was cursing the gift and God, closed the piano lid, stopped listening to concerts or music on the car radio, stopped all singing and stopped believing in God.

By 1972, when the U&I club for cystitis sufferers was started, I was beginning to know how desperately my stage and letter-writing skills were needed in alerting patients to self-help. Press, radio and television, as well as doctors, were alerted to the need for change in treatments for cystitis and Candida. At that time I was also beginning to see a pinprick of light at the end of my own tunnel and found a little phrase ticking in my mind 'God works in a mysterious way His wonders to perform.' I wish He hadn't picked me, but it's clear that He did, so I have no choice but to write, counsel, lecture and sing.

My marriage finally ended in divorce in 1985. We were never able to sexually bond early on, and the fight for my health knocked the stuffing out of both of us. When more difficulties arose between 1975 and 1982, I ran out of fight and divorced him.

Sadness and tragedy are not mine alone. Millions of women have their own variations of my story. Hopefully theirs will be shorter because in the 1970s I helped to create a climate of self-help both in Britain and in the USA. The emergence of associations, articles and self-help books has heralded a new age of patient-doctor partnerships, and this is to be greatly encouraged.

As a thrush/Candida sufferer, you should by now have trust in me; as a doctor or nurse reading this, you should know that your patients will be in very good hands, as my approach to this common problem is well researched and practical.

What should we call this illness?

There is some confusion as to what this condition should be called. Here's a brief run-down of some of the terms used.

THRUSH?

This is the term most commonly used in Britain; women elsewhere tend to say Candida or Yeast Infection.

CANDIDA?

This is the shortened version of Candida Albicans; it's simply easier to say.

CANDIDA ALBICANS?

This is a yeast organism present on surface skin and in all moist internal membranes.

YEAST INFECTION?

This is the term most commonly used in America to describe an overgrowth of existing fungal organisms leading to infection.

MONILIA?

This is just another, rather old-fashioned name for Candida Albicans. It's rarely used these days.

CANDIDOSIS?

This is the condition caused by Candida Albicans.

CANDIDIASIS?

This describes very severe systemic (whole-body)Candida illness created by the presence of Candida Albicans.

SYSTEMIC CANDIDA?

A user-friendly way of saying that the thrush is severe and present at more than one site.

First known as Monilia, this was the fungus that was faintly viewable under early microscopes in the mid-eighteenth century. It was discovered in rotted-down vegetation, but because compound lens microscopes had not yet been invented it was not possible to see the details of the organism through simple lenses.

In fact, some further time elapsed before the first reliable medical descriptions were noted. A Latin name was felt appropriate because the organism was clearly seen as white and stringy and in ancient Rome, a senator's political power and status was announced by the wearing of a long, white tunic (the toga). In the 1920s,

Candida, together with Albicans, meaning 'white', was internationally adopted by scientists and doctors to put an end to the muddle over which of the many names should be chosen.

'Thrush' has probably been in extensive use as a name - both with doctors and the general public - for several centuries. Although it may have originated as a Danish term, the resemblance to the speckles on the breast of the song thrush could well have initiated the term. Samuel Pepys recorded in his famed Diary on June 17th, 1665:

'He hath a fever, a thrush and a hickup!'

Trust that canny observer to pinpoint the symptoms which many of us recognise as wholly accurate to this day!

Throughout this book, I will try to keep terminology appropriate to the context. For instance, we all clearly understand vaginal thrush, and also thrush of the mouth or throat, but when discussion centres at any point on the major organs or systems, I prefer to call it Candida. This is grammatically incorrect but at least it is the right organism. The condition itself is officially known as Candidosis, although we all tend to call it either Candida or thrush. It is all the same causative yeast infection. Yeast Infection is also commonly heard, but 'infestation' seems to me to be a better expression.

Whatever the trouble, an attack is being mounted upon our normal wellbeing by an invasion or upsurge of organisms. This attack upon the normal balance of our body components produces responses. Much like the ripples from a pebble thrown into a lake, these responses fan out, often involving far more of our body than can be imagined. So all the following terms - Yeast, Fungal infections or infestations, Thrush, Candida, Candida upsurge, Candida infestation and Systemic Candida - will be used at some point, but for our purposes they are all one and the same problem.

A short history of vaginal thrush

Some of the earliest civilisations were keen on what we now call gynaecology. Early manuscripts written in Hindu around 800 BC showed a good knowledge and practical demonstration of the female anatomy. Early laparoscopies, abortions and caesarean sections were undertaken with a range of 125 kinds of instruments. One particular Hindu manuscript lists twenty-four diseases, one section of which notes various discharges. According to symptoms, early pessaries made of wool or lint were soaked in appropriate herbal mixtures for vaginal placement. Douches of herbal infusions were propelled into the vagina by means of pig's bladders which were simply filled, inserted and squeezed until all the contents had been released.

The Greeks, even before Hippocrates in 400 BC, had temples of healing where priests and priestesses helped locals with health difficulties. Cleanliness, being a religious rite, was employed as a rite of good health and patients entering were made to bathe before examinations by the Holy Ones. Women could be seen by priestesses or midwife/nurse counsellors if they requested. The priestesses undertook intimate treatments such as pessary insertion, douching, fumigation, childbirth, abortion and so on.

Fumigation, particularly, had to be done on site because it involved using a burning house or kiln. From here, smoke would be precisely directed via pipes to the room above, where, using hollowed-out lead pipes or reed pipes, the fumes could then be directed into the vagina or even higher into the cervical canal and uterus.

If the discharge was felt to be uterine in origin, then irrigation of the uterus was performed, using pipes and reeds leading out of cow's or pig's bladders to direct distilled herbal fusions high into the uterus. Often the cervix was then plugged up with lint or wool which, with the patient lying prone, would then have time to soak into the lining of the uterus.

Vulval diseases were not given much space in these early times, perhaps because most diseases in women were thought to be of the uterus and were of interest because of childbearing considerations. In Greece in AD23-79 Pliny, a notable herbalist, was famed for success with women's diseases and complaints. Amongst other things, he used garlic, rue and ammi for uterine fumigation. For 'the white flux', he made ointments of rose petals or scandix, probably as much to mask the unpleasant odours as to cure the trouble.

Soranus, of the Ephesus region in Greece, living in the first century AD, wrote fourteen treatises on the diseases of women. He was, by all reports, a splendid physician, promoting cleanliness and birth control by local methods, such as rancid oil on linten knots and honey smeared profusely on the cervix or sponge plugs. He, too, used fumigation, but there were, unfortunately, frequent cases of vaginal or cervical burns caused by over-hot smoke!

Fumigation was practised worldwide, it seems, for uterine or vaginal problems until the Middle Ages. Fumes were of many kinds including charcoal, frankincense, cassia, spikenard or storax.

OTHER PRACTICES

In addition to the pessaries, fumigation and herbal installation by douching mentioned above, there were other forms of treatment:

- dry fomentation: a hot, soggy substance would be sewn into the bladder of a pig or cow and inserted into the vagina for a few hours while the heat dissipated;
- wet fomentation: ordinary hot water would be inserted by means of a bottle, earthen or bronze pot or a sponge;
- cautery: hot arrow heads, hot irons or even animal teeth or horns would be inserted to lance abscesses, burn erosions and remove polyps or nodules;
- massage was frequently used for pain relief and fatigue. The Chinese were using this method and herbs or acupuncture in 3000 BC;
- pessaries were initially modelled from wax and oily ointments and only began to resemble our modern-day products at the beginning of the twentieth century.

Little headway, other than by observation and case history, was made until early microscopes began to make differentiation of organisms in discharges possible in 1683. Around this time, several eminent scientists began to develop the simple-lens microscope, which allowed exciting views of day-to-day organisms. This all progressed slowly until in France, Louis Pasteur (1822-1895) became the first person to discover yeasts, which caused fermentation. He also discovered the bacterial relationship to infectious diseases.

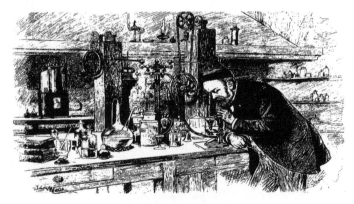

Louis Pasteur at work.

Vaginal discharges, however, remained largely undocumented. Variations of rmenstrual flows, gonorrhoea (the venereal disease) or leucorrhea (the normal, creamy female discharge)were the commonest discharges. All early societies documented these and offered remedies which may or may not have worked.

The first authoritative works specifically on thrush were only done with the help of simple microscopes. In 1839, Langenbeck in Germany reported the fungus following an autopsy he performed on a case of typhoid. In 1842, Berg in Sweden gave the first good, microscopic description and this excited Charles Robin in 1843 to investigate it carefully, naming it Oidium Albicans. Names for it subsequently changed frequently, as many medical papers were researched and written throughout the nineteenth century.

Intestinal thrush/Systemic Candida

Sadly, almost all early reports of thrush fail to mention the symptoms. There are certain works which, in passing, mention bloating, wind or odours, but it is hard to ascribe them directly to gut thrush, since the majority of books on intestinal or bowel disorders of early years are far more intent on the most basic medical discoveries, such as haemorrhoids, fistulas (lesions of the bowel), indigestion, gastroenteritis and what each part is called and what it does.

Because compound lens microscopes and the ability to culture secretions were not discovered until the last century, little was understood by physicians or surgeons of unreachable organs. They all did their best (or worst) provided it was possible to have reasonable access by pipes, reeds or fingers. Beyond this, they could not physically reach. Blood-stained mucus secretions appear to have interested doctors and writers most of all, so gynaecologists and obstetricians concentrated on childbirth and diseases associated with pregnancy, whilst early proctologists, who were interested in the bowels, were keen on bleeding haemorrhoids or pus-filled fistulas and abscesses.

Much of the rectal area (bowels) remained unknown until Professor Morgagni in Italy (1682-1771) decided to devote his life to naming and documenting it. However, when it came to Pruritis Ani (itching anus), it would appear that everyone either suffered from it or was seeing patients with it and, of course, it was easily visible.

The earliest mentions can be found on the Egyptian Papyrus scrolls of 3000 BC, referring to 'burning in the anus' and recommending suppositories of juniper, cumin, cinnamon, myrrh, honey or frankincense to 'expel the heat'. The vastly observant and experienced Roman writer Celsus, living in the reign of Emperor Augustus, noted a condition of 'anal cracks and pruritis ani - most tedious maladies'. He advised applications of hot, hard-boiled pigeons' eggs! Perhaps many cases of Pruritis Ani were due to worms, from which virtually everyone suffered continuously until very modern times.

This 'scourge' of doctors, proctologists and itchy patients was therefore well documented from earliest times and treated mostly, as previously mentioned, with suppositions or fomentations soaked in a variety of herbal distillations. However, surgery then became the fashionable way to treat almost every ill, barbarism crept in and terrible sufferings were meted out to already sick people. The coming of the Barber Surgeons in the seventeenth and eighteenth centuries took a hold on medicine until pharmaceutical discoveries, notably in the early twentieth century, restored the balance between surgeons and physicians.

With the advent of microscopes and work on the gastric contents of the stomach, it was possible at long last for Dr Blanchard in the USA to state in 1938 that Pruritis Ani was the result of fungal storage and upsurge. He had to hypothesise at first and battled against orthodox ideas of the day, which continued to use outdated surgical procedures to remove parts of the anus because they were thought to be secondary sites of cancerous mucus or pelvic disorders. Dr Blanchard argued aggressively that this was not so and that Pruritis Ani is the result of 'abnormal body chemistry and faulty digestion'. He was pretty well accurate in this. In additional case histories of patients, he was able to document intestinal bloating, wind, anal irritation and moisture 'as if the anus was bathed in perspiration'. He concluded also that 'barbarous surgical treatments ought to have been abandoned long ago'.

Instead, Dr Blanchard treated his patients with colonic irrigation, acidic dressings of diluted hydrochloric acid to clear the fungal infection and then followed up with soothing ointments. Pruritis Ani has been 'the bane of proctology', he said.

Digestion and intestines

Leaving the rectum and anus, it is of interest in this book to step back in time and acknowledge the start of our knowledge of intestinal contents.

One of the earliest known authors on this topic was Van Helmont in Holland (1577-1644) writing of 'an acid ferment'. He and his contemporaries spent much of the seventeenth century discussing digestion and how to find out what went on in the stomach and intestines. Birds and animals featured prominently in their attempts to find answers. Dead or alive, the poor creatures helped provide much early knowledge of secretions and mucus. Two most eminent scientists, Reanur in France and Spallinzi in Italy, wrote and experimented copiously, finding acidity, **fermentation**, alkalinity, **putrefaction** and neutrality of gastric juice. They sparked great international debates and prompted discoveries of many different stomach acids, including lactic acid, by Macquart in 1786. Dissent, argument and bad feeling were to be found in many laboratories as cascading works were done. By 1844, the basic truths were well in place, with discoveries of starch and sugar in the intestines. The discovery of the actions of salts, acids and crystals, fermentation processes, starch and **bacillus** organisms went on unabated into the twentieth century.

From those seventeenth-century experiments on birds and mammals, doctors finally moved on to humans in the nineteenth century. Many sick people gave up any semblance of comfort to submit to dreadful stomach-washing experiments and specimen collections so that knowledge could be obtained of gastric secretions. They must have been very frightened and in terrible discomfort, tied onto tables with their heads hanging over the edge whilst pints of water were pumped in and vomited out into collecting pails for analysis.

Finally, in the 1930s, the sheer size and scope of all these gastric discoveries rendered many of the medical observers lost, confused and exhausted. To their aid, in the early 1950s, came further advances in science and microbiology. Tests and experiments became much less arduous to conduct. There were some temporary gaps in the continuity of experiments, findings and write-ups in medical literature because of the two World Wars. Inevitably, medical concentration on fungal diseases took a back seat to war wounds, gangrene and gonorrhoea, which became epidemic. Men either died or were tremendously incapacitated as a result of 'sampling foreign delights'. Sexually transmitted to many wives and girlfriends, with obvious distress and resulting marital breakdowns, it took the discovery of penicillin by Sir Alexander Fleming for use in combating war-wound infections to establish it as a panacea for gonorrhoea too.

Inevitably, funding for this sort of research was far harder to find. The drug companies' capital outlays and reserves were directed almost solely into the research and production of drugs to help ailments more directly linked to the wars. Little manufacturing energy went into anything other than medications and supplies for troops or essential back-up services.

Post-war developments

The first post-war book on the subject, called Candida Albicans, was finally published in 1964, written by H.I. Winner and R. Huxley. A short time later, in the USA, Dr Orian Truss also brought out a useful book, 'The Missing Diagnosis,' which was an account of Candida in general practice. Since then, much has been written about it mostly in terms of diet causing many sufferers to become weaker. My book deals with causes and is sparing on diet.

Unfortunately, doctors are less than knowledgeable or sympathetic to sufferers since medical training teaches about athlete's foot, oral thrush of babies' being breastfed, Candida in HIV Aids and during the death process. Women find themselves being prescribed vaginal pessaries or occasional oral treatments but no real medical knowledge of the cause. They can fall victim to the trend of the last thirty years to depend on the prescription pad. Generic medicines (i.e. the basic drugs, as against brand names) always appear cheaper but can be more expensive if the patient fails to respond completely. Generic prescribing can be false finance, never mind the extra months of continued distress, anxiety, medical consultations, discomfort and general loss of wellbeing suffered by the patient

Dr James Papez, 1883-1958, sometime professor of Neuroanatomy in Cornell University, spent years investigating at autopsies, brains of deceased mental patients from a large mental institution of 2600 beds in Columbus, Ohio. He had begun observing living organisms from one chance brain encounter and moved into a series lasting seventeen years researching them. From obvious gum disease in these patients he was able, in autopsy, to trace the identical fungal organisms from gums to heart, brain, sclerotic patches and brain tumours.

Under microscope, various drugs were tried upon the fungal organisms: Serpasil, Thorizine, Aspirin and Phenetidin killed them but antibiotics did not. He classified them as the genus of Fungi Imperfecti with 21 varieties and called them Zoospores because they were very elemental in appearance often without the normal fungi attributions like stems or myelium. From his microscope specimens, Papez' wife drew beautiful illustrations to match his writings. The commonest one, Fungi Nigricans easily adapted to gums, cold sores, toe-nails, gingivitis, nerve cells, adrenal glands, prostate gland, digestive ulceration, blood vessels and many other sites. Nigricans and others were found to be episodic in upsurges rather than permanently acute. It is interesting that patients with heart disease today are advised to take Aspirin on a daily basis to increase arterial flow!

Papez found that their toxic enzymes attack proteins and fats causing fat globules to form in culture and that this action removed cell hydrogen causing carbon deposits. Under microscope he could clearly see that most body tissues were invadable by Zoospores from gum diseases and caused much ill health particularly in the brain where all manner of mental illness from nervousness to schizophrenia were backed by hospital case notes.

Such mycotic spores dissolve tissue very easily by draining the cell of life force and replacing it with toxic enzymes. This action was clearly seen in bone marrow where they formed granulated leukocytes also in granulated muscle fibres of the heart. In blood vessels granules form the cuffs of arteriosclerosis. In all these and other organs toxic enzymes replace healthy tissue and by further absorption cause nerve fibre reactions.

In 1951, new staining techniques in the laboratory enabled more detailed observations. Abundant mycotic spores were observed in the brains of all the mentally ill patients who were his source of available tissue and from this time, he worked tirelessly on linking fungal infestations of the jaw to mental and systemic illnesses. In 1957, Dr Papez accepted 50 granulated peridontal and alveolar specimens from crown and Root Canal Treatments for analysis and Report, all of which were found to match the patients' reported systemic illnesses when later revealed.

Peridontal abscesses contain these mycotic spores and spread to lymph, nerves and blood taking ill health everywhere including brain senility, heart disease, diabetes, hypertension and a host of others.

'Mycotic spores take possession of many human organs', Papez said.

Sourced: Ontario Dental Association Journal. March 1962.

Journal of Nervous and Mental Diseases. Vol. 119 No 4, April 1954.

The PAMA Compilation, 2002, for victims of mercury poisoning.

One thing is clear. We must take more responsibility, in the light of greater knowledge, for our own health. We must question ourselves and our doctors; we must search for answers amongst the health sections in bookshops and libraries. If you don't know something and your doctor is unhelpful or short of time, go and find out from Help lines, leaflets, books, counsellors, magazines, TV/radio, Health Authorities. Help will be out there waiting for you, but it won't walk into your sitting room uninvited! Never before in medicine or public health has there been such a balance between the professional and the patient.

> *Without the patient there would be no physician.*
> *Therefore the patient stands in priority to the physician.'*
> **Dr Delmer Davis, MD California, USA (1938)**

Many patients' knowledge on Candida already outstrips that of their doctor. Of course, if doctors keep abreast of the condition, then a true liaison can develop, but currently, this seldom happens. I hope that professionals who know of my pioneering work on cystitis, will now take advantage of my efforts in this book on Candida. It, too, is well researched, conventional and practical. So read and learn. We patients need you!

2 The base site - the digestive system

All detective stories have a location where the crime takes place. This book is a detective story, one based on known medical facts but where most of the policemen (doctors) and victims (patients) have failed to join up the clues, reach proper conclusions (diagnoses) and effect an arrest (cure).

The original venue for the crime of Candida upsurge is the gut. It is here that bacteria and yeasts combine in daily warfare to repel each other and maintain a balance (rather like the prevailing political attitudes during the Cold War - you launch one at me and I'll send mine back, with interest!).

Any good detective needs to get to know the characters involved and what happened at the scene of the crime. Knowledge of the venue is vital; so is knowledge of how the suspects arrived there and whether the offence was meditated or happened by chance.

We, as the victims of Candida, need a briefing on all this: so, too, do the doctors whom we visit so frequently in our distress. It isn't enough to take down a note of the incident, write the pessary prescription and forget it. Victims of an incident want action. We want the investigation and capture of the culprit and a full picture of the events as they unfolded. Satisfaction and closure are necessary, and there is no reason why, with current medical knowledge, they should not be possible.

Candida is dreadfully commonplace and is getting worse for all sorts of reasons. Like figures for cystitis, numbers for Candida infestations remain unrecorded, yet the costs of consultations, medications, social and sexual de-stabilisation are astronomical. The whole situation is unsatisfactory for everyone.

Investigating the crime

We are going to start our full investigations at the scene of the crime, the digestive system. Once we have been reminded of the physiological settings, we shall look at **micro-organisms** which inhabit this system and what functions they serve, where they come from, how they breed, what makes them occasionally disturbed and why all this links with Candida.

THE MOUTH

No matter what size it is, whether it belongs to birds, fish or mammals, its prime function is to take in food as energy for the body. As coal is to a fire, so food is to the body, a giver of life and energy. Nature works efficiently with gravity so that the whole process of digesting food uses an inner mechanism of muscle contractions rippling downwards.

In most species, the mouth can also be used as a weapon for attack or defense, but humans tend not to use this facility; we usually only use the mouth for eating, talking or kissing - not biting!

Physiologically, the mouth cavity starts at the lips, includes teeth and jaws and ends at the root of the tongue. Only the lower jaw moves: the upper jaw and hard palate (roof) are immobile. Elsewhere, the mouth is a mass of muscles covered with a mucus membrane which is always wet, but which becomes wetter when stimulated by food and drink. As we eat, we chew (or masticate) so that salivary glands are stimulated to provide enzymes and lubricants. Enzymes immediately begin to work on the food and break it down. Chewing also does this. Between the two actions, smaller pieces of food move to the back of the mouth waiting for the first big muscular contraction of the pharyngeal larynx (a swallow). The food is swallowed down into the gullet. The more chewing we can do before swallowing, the better. If we don't allow the mouth to function fully in the digestive process, we place greater strain on the stomach and intestines later on, since they have to deal not only with larger pieces of food but also reduced enzyme activity which would have helped break down the chunks.

When healthy, the mouth is clean and moist, but during illness it can become dry. Bacterial balance within the cavity can be thrown and, as with a sore throat or cold, bacterial invasion may occur. Fungal invasion also happens here for a variety of reasons which will be covered later. The mouth receives food of all sorts (again discussed later) and inhaled substances which dry out or contaminate the membranes. Oral health and hygiene can be paramount to the rest of our system. Bad teeth can mean a bad body, and bad food can result in a bad stomach.

THE GULLET (OESOPHAGUS) AND WINDPIPE (TRACHEA)

The gullet is linked to the mouth by the pharynx; as a 'swallow' develops, the oesophagus catches the food. Much like the open mouth and muscular ripples that can be seen in nature documentaries about snakes, so our gullet ripples food safely downwards with help from gravity. Its sole job is the conveyance of food, drink and excess mucus from mouth or nose.

The trachea is a long organ attached to the larynx. Inhaled air from our nose or

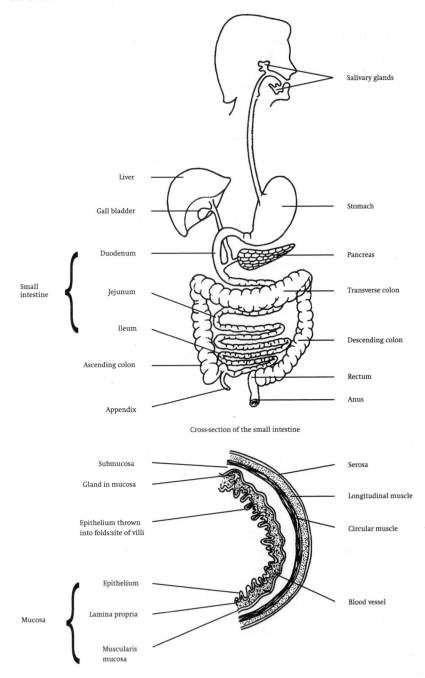

Salivary glands

Liver

Gall bladder

Duodenum

Small intestine

Jejunum

Ileum

Ascending colon

Appendix

Stomach

Pancreas

Transverse colon

Descending colon

Rectum

Anus

Cross-section of the small intestine

Submucosa

Gland in mucosa

Epithelium thrown into folds:site of villi

Mucosa

Epithelium

Lamina propria

Muscularis mucosa

Serosa

Longitudinal muscle

Circular muscle

Blood vessel

mouth becomes separated from food at the junction of the pharynx and larynx, and each is diverted down the appropriate pipe. The trachea lies in front of the oesophagus but whereas that organ transports its contents downwards (except during vomiting), the trachea has two distinct jobs. Firstly, it must carry air to our lungs, but secondly, it acts as a sentinel in seeking and trapping any mucus particles which, if allowed into the lungs, would interfere with easy breathing. So the trachea has a fine lining of 'cilia' which wave upwards towards the larynx and enable the cough mechanism to return whatever it was to the mouth. Here it will be swallowed correctly down the oesophagus and lung capacity will be safeguarded. Excess mucus from a cold, rhinitis, bronchitis or pneumonia is also expelled upwards by coughing.

THE STOMACH

The stomach is a multi-purpose bag, looking something like a bagpipe, whose sole purpose is the breakdown of large pieces of food. It has a formidable array of instruments at its disposal to achieve this. It can distinguish coffee and a piece of cake from a large meal and then employ different methods to use its machinery in the most effective and prudent way. Cake and coffee is easily liquified, so it is quickly passed out of the stomach into the duodenum and small intestines. For a meal, though, the passage into the duodenum is delayed until the full food-blender process has been turned on. Food is churned backwards and forwards, round and about by muscular contractions (for the stomach is, in reality, a great bag of strong muscles). Into the churning food mass goes a raised amount of digestive liquids which continue to break down the beaten-up food. If this has not been chewed up sufficiently well in the mouth, then the stomach has to make up for our laziness by extra activity, extra secretion of gastric juices. If the meal was very large two or more courses - we feel bloated, heavy, restless and find sleeping unpleasant if we have eaten at night. Our stomach feels likewise! The churning action is then very limited; fill up your food processor too much, and it takes longer for food at the top of the processor to find its way down to the blades!

Over-eating overtaxes all the stomach's skills and is generally not a good idea! To deal with too much food, gastric juices and gastric bacteria of all sorts have to multiply fast in minutes to help the digestion or breakdown of all these food particles. It has to be done; food cannot be expected to stay permanently in the stomach and, of course, it doesn't.

THE INTESTINES

In all, the length of the small intestine and the large intestine measures about twenty five and a half feet!

Small Intestine

This begins with the duodenum (the part of the small intestine which exits the stomach); it is roughly ten inches long. As well as continuing the process of breaking down food, the small intestine produces its own extra secretions (and others from the liver and pancreas) to liquidise the food particles still further. Further muscle rippling (peristaltic waves) carries the liquids along to the jejunum, which runs for about eight feet on to the third section of the small intestine, the ileum, completing its entire twenty feet. The one-and-a-half-inch width of this tubing is all muscle, and the inner surface is covered with tiny, brush-like hairs called 'villi'. These absorb the now-liquid food and pass it into capillaries of the bloodstream for use in energising the entire body. A meal, now liquified, passes through these twenty feet of small intestine in a few hours, but remaining, unusable food is passed into the large intestine.

Large Intestine

Here, from the ileum, liquids and remaining solid particles enter the colon where a vast array of bacteria is now set loose to start forming faeces. Faeces are waste products from the whole digestive process. Bacteria work at breaking down and reforming these rejected particles into faeces and are harmless whilst occupied with this function. About five feet long, the large intestine ends in the rectal cavity, the rectum, where sufficient faeces then stimulate the rectum to pass them out of the anus, a strong, muscular valve, to the outside.

THE PANCREAS

This is a hard-working gland which primarily aids digestion by controlling and alkalinising the acids in stomach juices. Secretions from the pancreas enter the duodenum, together with bile juice from the liver, from one shared opening and act there to neutralise excess acids as they emerge from the stomach and enter the small intestine. The pancreas secretes a hormone, insulin, which controls cellular ability to take glucose from the bloodstream after digestion.

THE LIVER

This is a large receptacle for blood which has been newly filled with nutrients from the digestive process. Cells in the liver receive, clean, store and send blood off to needy organs and tissue all round the body. The liver also secretes bile juice to the duodenum to further aid digestion, particularly of fats.

Thus the various organs of the alimentary canal (the digestive system) form the base site inhabited by Candida. Now we need a run-down of inhabitants, both natural inhabitants and those which invade or upsurge. Food ingestion is taken for granted; what we now need to know are the names and functions of the major components involved in the liquifying processes taking place at various points along the alimentary canal.

SALIVA IN THE MOUTH

This is the first liquid to combine with any food or drink. It is secreted from three sets of glands spread around the mouth. It does two jobs:

- keeps the mouth moist and clean by maintaining a bacterial balance;
- uses its enzyme, ptyalin, to begin breaking down starch in the food.

The more we chew at this initial phase of digestion, the more effective the whole digestive process will be. It breaks starch down into small molecules which the intestine finally converts to simple sugar. If we don't chew sufficiently, subsequent parts of the digestive process have an increased workload in order to compensate.

GASTRIC JUICES OF THE STOMACH

These are immensely strong and primarily acid. The stomach has to protect itself from them so a thick lining of the immensely powerful muscular wall secretes a protective membrane of alkaline mucus. When the stomach is devoid of food, gastric juice is minimal, but when food is swallowed, the combination of the volume, together with the nerve supplies, creates an outpouring of sufficient juice to digest that particular amount. About two litres of gastric juice a day are necessary to keep up average daily production. In the juice are scores of components about which whole books have been written. However, just for now, the main ones are:

- hydrochloric acid: provides appropriate levels of acidity and disinfectant defence against bacterial invasions;
- pepsin: helps digest proteins;
- amino acids: found in proteins and needed for absorption and good health;
- bicarbonate and other alkalines: keep the acidity levels under control;
- mucoproteins: encourage mucus production to protect the stomach lining;
- gastrin: a hormone which encourages secretion of acids and water;
- intrinsic factor: a secretion aiding vitamin B12 absorption lower down in the small intestine;
- volatile fatty acids (including lactic acid): have several jobs which help to balance alkalinity;
- enzymes of all sorts: help reduce particles of food and aid absorption.

INTESTINAL SECRETIONS, BACTERIA AND GASES

As we know, the function of the small intestine is to absorb prepared nutrients which are those minerals, salts and vitamins now swilling around in the liquified food called **chyme**. The villi (tiny hairs) dip into this liquid and absorb all good material, passing it in turn to the bloodstream. Within the small intestine, further decomposition and fermentation occur. These processes are made possible by the following:

- fermenting acids, including lactic acid, succinic acid, caproic acid, caprylic acid and acetic acid;
- yeasts of all sorts: these help fermentation and breakdown of food bulk;
- bile juice from the liver, comprising salts formed from cholesterol which perform a variety of functions: they mix with fat molecules in an emulsified liquid to make the fat more digestible; they enhance vitamin absorption (vitamin molecules A, D and K are poorly absorbed and wasted if amounts of bile salts are too low); they release other enzymes for digestion use. In addition, bile carries excessive cholesterol away to the duodenum for waste dispatch in faeces. All this activity puts the liver's output of bile juice at around a litre a day;
- pancreatic juice from the pancreas. This is alkaline and neutralizes acidity in the duodenum with bicarbonate secretions. Other contents called enzymes, enable food particles to become microscopic so that the capillary blood vessels can collect them for dispatch to organs and muscles. Chemical control of the balance of blood sugar levels is achieved by the hormone insulin. Glucogen, the second hormone released by the pancreas, encourages release of tissue sugar back into the bloodstream, mainly sugar stored in the liver;
- gases, including hydrogen, nitrogen and carbon dioxide;
- bacteria: there is not much bacteria to be found in the small intestine, but numbers increase towards the middle and then abound from the colon downwards into the large intestine. Here, they work at decomposition and fermentation. The more liquid food they receive, the more they respond by increasing their own numbers very quickly to continue their work and thus they continue to thrive. Undigested carbohydrate starch and glucose particles lying in the large intestine ferment, creating gases, acids and further breeding grounds. Numbers of bacteria are incredible. Eight grams of bacterial residue isolated from twenty-four grams of faeces produce 128 trillion bacterium.

Much bacteria is killed or controlled in the large intestine. Yeasts live or die according to the presence of an acceptable environment containing enough supplies both of dead bacteria and glucose. In many books on the digestive system, the dangers of insufficient chewing and of large meals are clearly emphasised:

'Adults who have no accurate knowledge or clear conception of the requirements of the body and who, either from a love of eating or from habit, overtax their digestive organs by over-eating or by flooding them with wine and beer, and who thus fill the lower portions of the intestines with fermentative and decomposing material suffer, as do young children, from "deleterious residues of food" in the intestine.'
D.W. Fleiner, Austria, 1910.

Symptoms of overeating include flatulence, bloating and disagreeably smelly gas.

BOWEL MUCUS

This carries a great deal of waste, since the rectal cavity (bowel) constantly fills up with faeces emerging from the large intestine. Faeces touch the moist, blood-laden, slippery, muscular walls of the rectum and can deposit bacterial or fungal residue. Normal, un-irritated rectal mucosal lining is pale pink but, nearing the anal opening, it becomes red because of the supply of blood vessels. An efficient, strong sphincter valve opens under faecal and muscular pressure to allow faeces out.

Invasion and upsurge of Organisms in the large intestine

The stomach and duodenum (right through to the upper part of the ileum) are almost devoid of organisms, mostly because gastric juices, doing their job properly, destroy them.

Intestinal colonization by organisms commences across the placenta (umbilical cord) during pregnancy into the developing foetus. Once born, further organisms from breast milk are passed directly from the mother's own digestive system into the infant's mouth. Before the infant progresses to solids, encouraging and activating full gastric juice production, many organisms slip by and start to colonise the small intestine.

In 1948, a Danish physician, Hans Gram, devised the first reliable way of classifying the array of bacteria being constantly discovered. By staining the slides upon which he had placed bacteria for observation, he was able to discover two groups which reacted differently to dyes; they became known as Gram (positive) and Gram (negative).

These two groups of bacteria proliferate in the intestines (once past the ileum); the two groups can be further broken down as follows:

- Gram negative (rod-shaped) **anaerobic** organisms:
  bacteroid fragilis
  bifidobacterium aduloscentis
  eubacterium narofaciens
  escherichia coliform
  streptococcus viridans
  streptococcus salivarius
  lactobacilli
- Gram positive organisms:
  streptococci of various kinds
  aerobic lactobacilli of various kinds
  fungi of various kinds

In faeces, the commonest groups of waste organisms discovered during laboratory culture are:

- anaerobes;
- lactobacilli;
- coliforms;
- yeasts.

All microscopic organisms are able to swim because of tiny, hairlike oars (flagellae) so they obviously need a moist environment to facilitate this. Some like to attach themselves to the mucus lining of the intestines where nutrients are always to be found. Intestinal villi constantly dip into the liquid chyme to absorb useful energy and protein particles which makes this lining very agreeable to organisms.

DIETARY BALANCE

The reproductive and support systems of these organisms automatically regulate numbers, though this is all dependent upon living and breeding requirements remaining constant. If the balance of these requirements is removed or disturbed, organisms literally fight each other off the precious sustenance that remains. If someone eats a high-carbohydrate, high-sugar, low-fat diet, yeast colonies increase in size to cope with the extra work in breaking down the sugars which also serve as their own food. Other bacteria start to lose the fight and decline in numbers, causing an organism imbalance. If the diet is returned to a better all-round balance, yeasts slowly decrease in numbers and allow other organisms to grow once more. This can take three months. If yeast overgrowth is restricted or killed by anti-fungal drugs orally administered, then there is faster restriction, though the remaining poorly balanced diet will, if not corrected, re-stimulate yeast overgrowth.

AMOUNT OF FOOD

Another serious factor in colony strength with resulting organism upsurge is the 'resting' time of excessive food intake from too much of one sort of food or large meals. Although food is liquified into chyme and has a lot of small intestine to travel through, by the time it reaches the end about twelve hours later, much of the water content has been drawn off by absorption into the villi.

This means that solids (i.e. early formation of faeces) have begun to take shape. Sometimes, part of this residual waste from excessive amounts of one food or too much food actually hangs around in the colon for a week or so. Lack of exercise, amount of food eaten, laziness of clogged-up peristaltic waves moving waste along the large intestine, will all combine to encourage micro-organisms to breed and upsurge above their normal limitations.

DIARRHOEA AND CONSTIPATION

Diarrhoea loses good nutrients, organisms and liquid too fast causing dehydration and weakness. Constipation will do the reverse by straining the whole digestive system. Organisms upsurge, haemorrhoids swell and yeasts in particular thrive on the putrefaction and gases produced by this. Symptoms may include lethargy, fever, bloating, wind and weight gain.

Constipation can be caused by

- a large meal (two or three courses);
- insufficient exercise;
- too many binding eggs per week (two is the standard dietary advice);
- too much white, refined rice (experiment for individual levels);
- too much red meat (twice a week is acceptable in small amounts);
- too much white sugar and flour (wean off these to almost nothing);
- too much bran (wheat clogs the colon ridges - oatmeal is better).

Constipation may also occur if colonic intrinsic and enteric nerve systems are damaged or weakened by disease or accidents. These nerve systems are linked to the lumbar spinal column, so people paralysed or injured in that region will probably not be able to open their bowels without some kind of stimulus. Manual evacuation of bowels may become a daily essential for them. Conversely, walking is a great stimulant to a regulated bowel evacuation.

Peristaltic wave movements in the intestines continuously propel liquids and particles along. If they cannot accomplish this job, the intestinal part of the digestive system slows, becomes sluggish, and organisms will have to increase in numbers to cope. As they activate and work, yeasts have time to multiply too.

GASTRO-INTESTINAL GAS

Those of us who have experienced Candida upsurges will recognise only too well what 'gas' means. It means great embarrassment from stomach gurgles and burping to holding back - with some pain - a large fart in a public place and passing copious amounts of offensive wind in private. Stagnant gas manufactured during the long hours of sleep bursts forth upon awakening. It may not stop until after breakfast, when additional food and drink has nudged it further along.

This gas comprises carbon dioxide, hydrogen, oxygen, methane and nitrogen, which make up roughly ninety-nine per cent of a good fart! Its smell is caused by the other one per cent - a mixture of ammonia, hydrogen sulphide, skiatole and explosive amines. Gas arrives in the intestines from the air we breathe, the food we eat, drinking and some via the bloodstream but most gas found in the intestines and rectum is caused by bacterial fermentation.

FERMENTATION

Fermentation is also caused by:

- bicarbonate, sugars and yeasts, both indigenous intestinal flora and through reactions with chyme and indigestible foodstuffs. Enzymes aiding absorption and digestion either work harder or fail to work on things like cabbage, sprouts, onions, broccoli, nuts, prunes, plums, cauliflower and others, Gas results;
- Excessive glucose from sugars and fruits, which become unused and are stored or passed out as waste. It serves to support bacterial and yeast growth in the colon and intestines;
- alcohols and vinegars, which are already fermented products and are friendly to yeasts already colonised in the intestines;
- rotting vegetation, which causes bubbles of warm gases to rise, aided by the addition of sugar as food to the yeasts and bacteria, which require energy to cause the fermentation process;
- sugar, yeasts, flour and water when making bread. These create the bubbles that make it rise into dough;
- hops, malt, sugar, yeasts and liquid which form the light, airy, gaseous brew when beer is made.

These are all results of the process of fermentation. Our intestinal contents ferment on a regular basis normally; it is abnormal amounts of fermentation that predispose so many millions of us to Candida upsurge.

Yeasts and moulds

Yeasts of all kinds are derived as fungi. Yeasts are able to cause fermentation when mixed with sugar and liquid. They also like warmth and darkness. Yeasts are living cells from living plants, which become airborne in wind or waterborne from a rain shower, so that either the force of wind or rain can deposit the cells upon soil. So we can find yeasts in air, water and soil. You do not have to have an overactive imagination to see that human beings breathe, drink and eat yeast cells permanently. They live in our intestines.

Budding formation

Wherever yeasts are found, in water, soil, air or the intestines, so will also be found bacteria. The two are inextricably linked. For example, soil contains bacterial residue from animal and human faeces, yet we see no evidence of diseases on that spot of ground or anywhere around it. The soil copes because plants give off yeast cells which want their own 'space' to thrive. They are not willing to let bacterial deposits take over. So battle between the two is permanently joined and a natural balance occurs. Additionally, in earth, the drying action of sunlight helps remove water which both bacteria and yeasts have to have to survive at all. However, in human and animal intestines, there is no sunlight. They are permanently moist and dark; there is a permanent supply of both bacteria and yeasts and there is a permanent supply of sugar and alcohol - ideal conditions for breeding.

These fundamental observations were begun by Selman Waksman in the 1930s and addressed to the National Academy of Sciences in Washington in 1940. Waksman was the first scientist to use the term 'antibiotic' to describe an agent - mould or yeast working to kill bacteria. Until the late 1930s, it had been termed 'antibiosis'. He obtained the first dose of streptomycin from fungal organisms known as streptomycetes in 1943. The first works published on fungi came out in the 1920s and 1930s, although even in 1896 crystals were obtained from moulds of the penicillin family. However, it was not until a team of scientists in England developed purification techniques of moulds that clinical production for human use began in 1938.

Moulds, or fungi, were easily the most widely used antimicrobial sources of early pharmaceutical endeavours to kill bacterial infections. In other words, scientists tried to harness the natural combat between bacteria and yeasts in creating antibiotics- anti life. Today several of our highly developed antibiotics are derived from mould cells. Much purification takes place, but apparently no mould finally enters the body during a course of antibiotic treatment. That may be so now, but in the 1960s and 1970s, could mould (fungi) genetics have slipped through the manufacturing processes and be 'born again' once in the intestinal mucus?

If so, despite medical denials, could this be another possible explanation for the high modern incidence of Candida upsurges following antibiotic therapy? We have always understood Candida and other yeasts to be opportunists, upsurging when other sets of bacteria are occupied with an incoming illness. But what if there are also additional mutant moulds being newly placed within the intestine by drugs? I am assured by several pharmaceutical scientists that this simply cannot happen.

Most of the modern findings on yeasts have been made since the ending of World War II and during the 1950s. This is because of better microbiology facilities, in turn helped by better funding. Pharmaceutical companies, ever ready to spot market influences, could not fail to spend time and money on the new opportunities afforded by patients who were now being 'fed' antibiotics for virtually any infection by many doctors. Investment and scientific research was strongly encouraged to discover anti-yeast/fungal medications; in fact, they represented a whole new source of profitable medications and drug company income.

So, in 1959, Hasenclever and Mitchell were the first microbiologists to divide the many species of Candida Albicans into groups A and B when certain tests were done on them in the laboratories. Over 150 types of Candida exist as known today, and I do not intend listing them all here, but precise tests do exist if requested by the doctor. It is useful to know some of the commonest strains of Candida:

• Catenulata	• Krusei	• Glabrata	• Stellatoidea
• Kefyr	• Guilliermondii	• Tropicalis	• Claussenii
• Famata	• Lusitaniac	• Parapsilosis	

There are dozens of other Candida species, but we will not dwell on them here. A great deal of work is still in progress around the world on Candida; strains and subtypes, chromosomes and nuclei, DNA development strain to strain, colony formations, colony sites, cell shapes. As fast as one question is answered, a dozen more arise.

WHAT DOES CANDIDA LOOK LIKE?

It looks like buds - yes, just like the tiniest, early rosebuds appearing in our gardens around May. But these tiny buds, invisible to the naked eye, have broken away from yeast cells. If such a bud finds a pleasant spot in our intestines and has a good supply of converted sugar, it may grow strongly. It can grow in stringy shapes or convivial groups. At certain stages, when full of growth energy, other spores (buds) may form and break away. It's a constant multiplication process aided by its environment and the availability of food. The outer edge of a Candida bud is tough and resilient, changeable and able to attach itself to intestinal mucus, almost like Velcro. Candida buds can also form long filaments which act like Velcro adherent and are called hyphae.

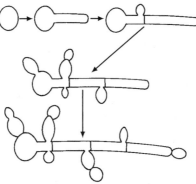

Hyphae formation

WHERE ELSE DOES IT LIVE?

Remembering that we commonly breathe it in and eat it, we can expect to find normal amounts of it in our mouth, gullet, intestines, bowels and excreted faeces. This is quite normal. It can also be introduced into the bladder by contaminated objects such as catheters, hospital drips, finger nails, unprotected cutlery, an infected penis, contaminated syringes, the list goes on. Hygiene is the watchword.

Some Candida in the vagina is usually present as part of the normal flora, but abundant growth and subsequent discharge will most likely occur with candidal excretion from faeces. This contaminates the perineum (pelvic area) and travels into the vagina en masse. As it does this, contamination of the urethral opening and tube can occur simultaneously.

Once settled in mildly acidic bladder lining, Candidal cystitis can cause misery and frustration for many people.

Candida in faeces is abundant, not only during an upsurge in the gut. Normal colonies will adhere to E. coli, which also abounds as an intestinal bacterium, so, as peristaltic waves push and form faeces in the large intestine, Candida and coliforms together arrive at the rectum awaiting expulsion through the anus. Once out of there, additional breeding grounds await. The first is the vaginal epithelium (mucosal skin) to which Candida makes a beeline, fixing preferentially onto older cells which are past their prime. Then it spreads to labia, perineum,inside leg and bladder. Candida can also be carried in the bloodstream, having come across the intestinal villi and blood capillaries. Once there, the whole body bloodstream supports and carries it. This was first proven in 1930 and is now well accepted and researched, though blood samples are often negative and certainly expensive. A cheaper, more efficient, test would be welcome. Those species of Candida most likely to use this means of spreading are Candida Parapsilosis, Kefyr and Albicans, but they are not the only ones.

Candida usually fails to find a suitable home on any part of the body that is free from mucosal linings. Outer skin is dry and airy, not moist and dark. This outer skin also sheds cells by the million onto clothing, bedding and into the bath or shower; however, if the sufferer has a lowered immune system, gets frequently sweaty without appropriate daily showers and powdering and also has areas that irritate easily, Candida may perhaps find an external area of skin to colonise. If there is severe oral Candida of the throat and oesophagus, then the outer edges of the mouth may show scabs and lesions (cuts) where hyphal infiltration of moist lips further increases the infestation. Ears and nasal passages may also become involved.

Blood-borne Candida spores burrow into the innermost layers of skin (the dermis), where capillaries network. Under the skin, colonies form at will, and if these reached the surface skin (the epidermis), we would see a pink rash dotted with white spots, possibly advancing to nasty-cooking blackened scabs in extremely severe cases. This may occur on any part of the body.

Candida in the eyes was reported as long ago as 1943, but no work was undertaken, despite several other sightings, until 1969. This came about because several patients who had received eye surgery all became infested with Candida which had colonised from the air and contaminated fluids needed during the surgery. It seems that a compromised immune system is again heavily involved and that, once the whole body is vulnerable to systemic Candida, even eyes are not spared the spread of the disease.

In short, no part or organ of the body is secure from the ravages of systemic Candida. All these findings have occurred over the last twenty years and volumes are being written by scientists all over the world. Efficient, cheaper testing at general practice level is surely required. Patients, often more knowledgeable these days from health books and magazine articles, find it extremely hard to face up to a doctor who is not well versed in Candida. Other than self help which will be discussed later, prescribing of Candida-killing drugs can only be done by a doctor and we, as patients, need to be reassured that the right one is being prescribed!

WHAT DOES CANDIDA EAT?

It eats sugars in the form of glucose. Once sugars from any source in our diet are fermented and form acceptable sugar for bloodstream absorption, it becomes known as glucose. Digestion breaks down sugars from an enormous range of foods and drinks. Glucose occurs naturally in fruit, honey, potatoes and rice as starch, beer, ale, wine and mead.

Most commercial foodstuffs, even savoury, have added sugar. Candida ferments all this glucose, creating spores and gases as it does so. It also likes to assimilate carbon and nitrogen gases, and some oxygen, but doesn't need lots of vitamins or minerals. Outside our bodies, scientists have to devise other additional nutrients to encourage it to grow on the culture plates, so they add thiamin, biotin, vitamin B 12 and a few other things. We already have a good intestinal supply of such additions.

WHAT OTHER FACTORS ENCOURAGE IT TO OVERGROW?

A nice warm home! It hates cold or cool temperatures, although it may struggle to survive for a while. Of course, it favours our body temperature most of all, 37C, but it can also grow anywhere between 20 and 38C. This is a wide range, taking account of very sick people who may have 'hot' fevers, with elevated temperatures, or 'cold' fevers, where shivering and cold limbs also show a compromised immune system coping with illness. It prefers an alkaline medium, but will cope with mild acidity. One of the many laboratory failings in testing and culturing for Candida is the great inner complexity and amount of additional substances in the intestines. This scenario is impossible to recreate outside in a laboratory. Intestinal balance between all the micro-organisms is held only within those digestive organs and systems.

Scientists have years to go before a fully comprehensive knowledge of the interaction between various gut yeast species can be documented. However, it makes no sense to add to existing colonies by ingesting yeasty or fermented food substances. Dealing with the existing trouble is difficult enough without consciously sending down reinforcements. All yeast species are capable of overgrowth and may prove to be 'allies' in an encouraging environment.

WHAT FACTORS ENCOURAGE IT TO DIE?

Candida and other yeasts will never die out. This has probably become fairly clear from reading the book so far, though Professor Odds in his book Candida and Candidosis does query at one point whether every single person really does have a capacity for allowing colony growth. He wonders whether some people simply pass yeasts straight through or have sufficient ability to withstand their attempts to colonise intestinal mucosa.

Bacterial balance with yeasts seems to be a major control factor, but impossible to monitor, since we cannot 'see' into our intestines when we notice upsurges in very obvious places like the vagina or even increases in bloating and farting; this notification is several days down the production line of the original Candida upsurge. Lifestyle modifications to avoid known Candida causes are dealt with later in the book and they are hugely helpful in trying to maintain a reasonable balance of bacteria to yeasts, as well as helping the immune system.

Candida-killing drugs are also effective and will be discussed later, but they are in themselves very strong and not to be taken lightly. We know that Candida enjoys an alkaline environment, so an acidic one should therefore be likely to inhibit growth and discourage spore production. Bicarbonate is constantly produced in the stomach to counter acidic gastric juices and further production or secretions throughout the chyme's intestinal journey create profuse alkaline mediums. Candida upsurge would respond favourably to individual digestive systems where alkalinity tends to overbalance the acidity. Yet, wherever over-acidity occurs within the digestive tract, so alkaline secretions are produced to counter-balance. We do not appear to be able to win on this!

The more you get to know, the more you realise you don't know. No two people are alike in the fine detail either of their bodies or of their worth and value in close clinical research or trials. It may be many years before all the factors predisposing or causing yeast control can be discovered. Scientists, researchers, writers and readers are trying to place the rules and findings in some order, but understanding and control of Candida is a new field. It demands patience, vitality, inquisitiveness, tenacity and elements of chance or luck.

3 Glucose production and control

Given that the amount of ingested food dictates, to a certain degree, the amount of bacterial and yeast activity required to aid its digestion in the digestive system, and given that bacterial and yeast balance is a vital controlling factor, then we should take a look at the mechanisms controlling the uses, storage, breakdown and control of the favourite food of Candida - sugar.

I shall be dealing with sugar in the diet later, but here I want to look at the way our digestive system deals with it. Very simply put, it may well be that those sufferers of Candida who aren't diagnosed as diabetic may instead have some hiccup in the way that their digestive system, or chemistry, as we shall call it in this chapter, copes with sugar. Think of a jar full of preserves or jelly; it can only contain a precise amount for that particular jar - any extra just dribbles down the sides. Each of us is like that jar when it comes to coping with sugar. Any amount over the body's ability to assimilate and use it causes strain or overflow. The extra energy produced in the final product comes off as unpleasant and abnormal gases and illnesses.

These sugars, which I will look at in detail, feed Candida. It will be interesting to know how our chemistry copes, breaks down, utilises and expels sugar ordinarily. Once we understand something of this, we may be even clearer about the strains placed upon this chemistry when we eat more sugars than our system can manage. It may help to consider the various components of food.

Carbohydrates and sugars

Starch is the commonest form of carbohydrate and is found as a staple item in almost every diet worldwide. We know potatoes, rice and flour as carbohydrates, all of which come from plants. Carbohydrates from all plants begin as carbon, hydrogen and oxygen compounds - basic gases able to form into molecules of starch when mixed with water, carbon dioxide and energised by sunshine. Work on breaking down starch into glucose begins in the mouth and continues.

Most of our body energy is produced by breakdown of carbohydrate starch into energy. This is the type of energy we refer to when we say, 'He's full of energy' implying a level of vitality, alertness, motivation and activity. This can be very intense, as in sportsmen and women or dancers, or quite the opposite, in a seriously sick patient in bed. Our energy for living is derived from what we eat and from our ability to utilise foodstuffs to maximum advantage.

In different societies, the amount of energy derived solely from carbohydrates (as against fats and proteins) varies greatly. In poorer countries cheap, carbohydrate foods are used as sources of energy but poor people tend to eat less often and not much anyway. People in richer countries have ready access to more costly **proteins** and fats, from which a greater carbohydrate/fat protein balance is achieved. They eat larger portions and have more meals so keeping digestion processes constantly busy and strained.

There are several broken-down forms of carbohydrates:

- **monosaccharides**: one simple sugar molecule;
- **disaccharides**: two sugar molecules combined from cane sugar and sugar beet to form ordinary, household sugar. Another disaccharide is maltose, formed from the malting or fermenting of barley starch, and yet another is lactose, present as a sugar in milk;
- **trisaccharides**: combination of three sugars, like those in molasses, a very thick, brown liquid. Glucose, galactose and fructose form raffinose, which is the chief sugar of molasses;
- **hexoses**: formed from monosaccharides. An important alcohol section of hexose, found in rowan berries, is used as the sweetener for commercial diabetic, sugar-controlled foods like jam. This sweetener is called Sorbitol and can not only produce energy, but will, at the same time, manage to be absorbed without adding to bloodstream sugar levels, which are the big concern in diabetes.

GLYCOGEN

This is the animal form of starch. It is still a form of carbohydrate, but it emanates from animals, not plants.

GLUCOSE

Glucose is the result of chemical enzymes acting upon and changing starches, sugars, carbohydrates, proteins and fats into smaller particles. It is a pure, refined sugar that is the end product of digestion. It is this that our bodies use as energy. It is glucose that is fed in a drip to patients too ill to eat solids by mouth, but still requiring nutrition.

Fats, lipoids and oils

This is a big group and various other terms are linked with it.

- Fats are also termed 'triglycerides', since they are compounded with a substance called glycerol. Fats are usually acidic and are alternatively called 'fatty acids', amongst which we find stearic acid, oleic acid and palmitic acid. During digestion, they can become acetic acid. They are also important as an end-of-chain energy producer, since fermentation finally converts them into glucose too. Some fats and lipoids are stored as bulk in cells for insulation, but can always be released for energy if required.
- Lipoids are, like fats, unable to mix in a water-based solution, but the way in which body chemistry digests them is so like fats that they are linked with them. Cholesterol is a lipoid.
- Oils start out in liquid form like fish oil, dripping, olive oil and so on. They are used and broken down just like fats and lipoids.

Protein

This is taken in from eggs, fish, meat, cheese, dairy products and converted down the digestive, chemistry chain into amino acids. There are dozens of amino acids with a multitude of uses within the body, such as forming other proteins, making up weight in the muscles and tissues, producing energy, healthy cell function. The end resulting amino acid comprises carbon, hydrogen, oxygen, nitrogen and occasionally sulphur. The formation of individual amino acids into chains is a highly individual one and is part of DNA analysis (i.e. the discovery of genetic blueprints that dictate what each human, plant, animal, fish or reptile will be like).

Liquids

Foodstuffs contain liquids, but the primary source of body fluid is taken in as pure liquid drink. Water contains a variety of additives these days in order to cleanse and purify it, particularly in large cities where the Water Authorities re-use it from treatment works. Pure water supplies from springs contain useful minerals for the body, like magnesium, but manufactured drinks contain heavy sugar and additives. Seventy per cent of our body weight is water.

These, then, are the main groups of liquid and food substances fuelling and energizing us. The energy created by them allows us to walk, talk, reproduce and generally thrive. There are two other ingredients necessary in our diet, minerals and vitamins. Absence of them can create holes or hiccups in the smooth functioning of body chemistry processes. All sorts of diseases can be caused by vitamin and mineral deficiencies.

Minerals

Magnesium
Is identifiable for recovery from arteriosclerosis, palpitations, cramping limbs, weakened bones, PMT and other ailments. It is mostly stored in bone marrow and aids glucose control.

Calcium
Mostly found in bones and teeth. Lack of it is indicated in osteoporosis, weakened bones, muscle pains, gum recession and heart irregularity.

Phosphorus
Maintains energy and strength in tissue cells.

Potassium
Without sufficient potassium in the cells, blood sugar is less readily converted into glycogen. Blood sugar levels rise and force the pancreas to produce extra insulin. Diuretic drugs increase its loss in urinary output.

Sodium
Largely stored outside cells, but is finely balanced with potassium inside cells. Sodium attracts and stores water, often causing swollen feet and legs. In balance, it helps regulate body fluid levels.

Chlorine (chlorides)
Works very closely with potassium and sodium in fluid regulation.

Iron
Vital in energy protection. Lack of it causes anaemia (a low red blood cell count) with resulting lethargy and lowered resistance to infection.

Zinc

Important for enzyme stimulation in bones, tissues and the pancreas. It is also responsible for efficient breakdown of body alcohol. Symptoms of zinc deficiency include loss of taste, skin disease, loss of appetite, poor healing. Diets high in fibre can induce low levels of zinc. Refined flours and sugars cause zinc depletion. Allergic people usually have low zinc levels.

Copper

Helps enzyme activity throughout the body. Some stays in the brain, some in the liver and some in the muscles. Deficiency can cause rheumatic disorders in some people, though it is also a suspect in many other illnesses.

Manganese

Mostly stored in bones. Lack of it is partly responsible for a variety of diseases such as epilepsy, metabolic disorders, schizophrenia and possibly heart diseases. It aids glucose control, so manganese depletion may play a part in upsurges of Candida. Manganese inter-relates closely with Magnesium and Calcium.

Iodine

Lack of it is known to cause malfunction of the thyroid gland, which is where most iodine is stored.

ULTRA TRACE MINERALS

Selenium, Chromium, Molybdenum

All three are involved in enzyme stimulation and control of blood sugar levels.

Selenium acts as a mercury chelation agent and can be scarce in a body poisoned by mercury from teeth fillings. Take a Selenium supplement and it eases aching bones and joints because it is binding onto and ejecting some of the stored mercury. Chromium is necessary in insulin metabolism (see Diabetes chapter).

Vitamins

These are vital external components within foodstuffs. Vitamins are never manufactured within the body; like minerals, they have to be introduced at sufficient daily levels in order to assist metabolism of all kinds. Most encourage various enzymes to do their particular jobs, so a vitamin shortage may result in faulty enzyme reaction which, in turn, will lead to faulty chemical or hormone reaction, which produces a faulty digestion of one of the proteins, carbohydrates, fats, or sugars. If the final result means that digestion and energy have been improperly conducted, then we may feel in some way unwell. We may upset the balance between bacteria and yeasts.

We need a brief rundown of the major vitamins; brief is all it can be, since a full disclosure would mean a separate book!

Vitamin A

Also known as retinol. It is primarily an alcohol coming from animals and plants. Fat digestion may be impaired as a result of Vitamin A deficiency, since the two combine in bile juice secreted from the liver, with Vitamin A assisting fat absorption in the small intestine.

Vitamin B complex

Comprises a great many different components, all classified under the original B heading. Again, stimulating enzyme activity is prioritised. Although numbered as B, B2, B6, B 12, etc., names are also given. Vitamin B complex includes pyridoxine, folic acid, riboflavin, thiamin. Deficiency of the complex is common in heavy drinkers or those undergoing antibiotic therapy.

Vitamin C

Easily destroyed in cooking and comes from fruit and vegetables. Its infection-fighting properties were well defined by Dr Linus Pauling in the 1960s. Vitamin C is also known as ascorbic acid, and its other function is to form fibres connecting tissue to tissue throughout the body. It also chelates mercury.

Vitamin D

Helps to maintain healthy bones. It helps calcium to achieve its full potential in bone maintenance and reformation and comes from fish oils, eggs, butter and sunlight. I am against all fish products because of the inherent carriage of mercury (see mercury amalgam section).

Vitamin E

Helps in fat digestion. Helps restore damaged skin.

Vitamin K

The stimulant for an enzyme, thrombolin, which is instrumental in helping a bleeding cut or graze to clot. Absence of it causes continued bleeding. The action of bile juice is important to the absorption of Vitamin K in the intestine.

Enzymes and hormones

Enzymes have been mentioned a lot already and this next section will draw upon the enzymes involved in food breakdown. We will also look at aspects of sugar/starch breakdown.

WHAT IS AN ENZYME AND WHAT DOES IT DO?

An enzyme is a protein which, by using fermentation, acts as a catalyst between two substances to form another. This catalysis only requires tiny amounts of the enzyme to trigger the required action, but each enzyme only has one specific job to do. The thousands of enzymes that make up our body chemistry don't interchange jobs. There are also co-enzymes, which act as go-betweens for two separate enzymes, both having some dual role in a particular process. Co-enzymes can also be an initial stimulus to another enzyme, forcing it to do its job. Vitamins, as we have seen already, are essential for correct enzyme activity, and if they are deficient, vital enzyme activation of other chemical substances fails to occur and can lead to illness.

Enzyme engineering is a modern, manipulative science by which illness can be counteracted through interfering with enzyme activity.

Bacteria have inner enzymes which, when de-activated by drug action, cease to grow, thus allowing the patient to recover. Many drugs have enzyme interference as their basis.

In digestion, many important enzymes formed in the pancreas travel to the intestines to bring about the chemical changes needed to break down remaining food particles. They don't work in the pancreas itself; they only activate once they have met up with food in the small intestine. These pancreatic enzymes are:

- trypsin and hymotrypsin;
- pancreatic amylase;
- ribonuclease;
- carboxypeptidase;
- lipolytic enzymes (including lipase);
- elastases.

All of these - and many more - are involved in digestion of sugars, proteins, fats and carbohydrates within chyme. The basic pancreatic juice is richly bicarbonate and therefore alkaline.

WHAT IS A HORMONE AND WHAT DOES IT DO?

A hormone is a chemical substance produced by glands situated within any organ. Hormones are released into the bloodstream to travel directly to another specific organ where the action of that organ is influenced. There are hundreds of hormones operating in our bodies, each sending its own specific messages. Sometimes hormones act independently and sometimes they join up to send longer messages. Hormones associated with the pancreas are:

- secretin, which provides alkalinity for pancreatic juice;
- CCK (cholecystokinin), which controls release of pancreatic enzymes;
- insulin, which moves glucose into body cells from the bloodstream.

Insulin

Insulin was first discovered in 1921 by two researchers, Banting and Best, in Canada. In 1958, the Nobel Prize for chemistry was won by F. Sanger for documenting its precise formation. Too much insulin in the bloodstream causes hypoglycaemia by rapidly lowering sugar levels; too little insulin in the bloodstream allows excessive sugar levels to remain unused as body fuel because cells cannot absorb it. Excess sugars are then designated waste by kidney sifting, and travel to the bladder in urine. Diabetes, as the condition of having insufficient insulin is called, can be diagnosed from excessive glucose found in urine samples. Some of this excess sugar may have been utilised earlier by yeasts in the intestines, so diabetics have a constant battle with Candida, as well as trying to balance their blood sugar levels.

Even without an insulin problem, there is a limit to the ability of the pancreas to manufacture enough of it, quickly, to deal with sugar overload from ingested foods.

The human body has evolved over thousands of years in association with basic foodstuffs - berries, plants, vegetation, animals and natural sugars. These foodstuffs are all within the boundaries of successful digestion but modern commercial sugar additives put a huge strain on an unprepared digestive system. As yet, human digestive evolution has not improved our capacity to assimilate and digest these additives without side effects.

It is important to reiterate that our digestive system is entirely stimulated by the introduction of food and drink. Enzymes, hormones, organs, juices, glands, peristaltic waves, muscles, bacteria, yeasts, acids, alkalines and all the rest of it respond. If we overeat, we cause chaos - some things speed up, some overgrow, some slow down, some become strained; we can be the personal authors of this, so we should think carefully about craving and bingeing!

WHAT ROLE DOES THE LIVER PLAY IN DIGESTION?

The liver is a gland, the largest gland we have. It receives blood from the capillaries of the intestines packed with usable sugars, proteins and fats in their various broken-down forms. It is also connected to the duodenum so that bile juice can flow from a sub-structure, called the gall bladder, to aid digestion.

Without a working liver, we would die. Amongst its vital jobs are:

- aiding digestion through the production of bile juice which is rich in enzymes and hormones;
- redistributing proteins and other nutrients;
- storing glucose as in glucogen;
- combating invading substances injurious to health, e.g. alcohol.

The liver is a highly complex gland and performs many other functions. However, from our point of view, its major role is as a storage and carrier vessel of glucose, which feeds yeasts.

A great deal of body chemistry occurs in the liver, and we have only scratched the surface here; suffice to say that, for the study of Candida, it is important to know that the liver is closely involved with sugars.

GLUCOSE USE AFTER DIGESTION

Following digestion, glucose is formed, regulated by insulin and stored in the liver. Excess is excreted via the kidneys into the bladder and then out as a component of urine. Our need for glucose is as a fuel to provide energy for movement and warmth.

HOW DOES GLUCOSE CAUSE MUSCLE MOVEMENT?

Just above each kidney lies a gland called an 'adrenal'. From the adrenal glands, which control part of the sympathetic nerve system, two hormones are secreted: adrenalin and noradrenalin.

Adrenalin

Through a chemical activity, this hormone releases glucose out of the bloodstream into tissue. Much of this tissue is muscle, used in movement. Muscle cells absorb glucose to satisfy their own energy requirements. These trillions of micro-cells, acting together under instruction from the brain, then continue to create whatever movement has been requested - walking, talking, writing, lifting.

Noradrenalin

This is concerned mainly with blood pressure.

Other hormones are also secreted from another section of the adrenal glands. These, too, have a role to play in glucose tissue absorption. Between them, cortisone and aldosterone regulate the storage and usage of glucose, sodium and potassium, all three being used by tissue cells for muscle movements. Cortisone and aldosterone are part of a group of hormones termed cortiscosteroids. These are essential for all sorts of body chemistry processes, such as inflammation, fat regulation and distribution, allergic responses, keeping stress levels tolerable, heart stimulation and others.

Adrenaline, for example, is not just adept at preparing muscles for movement through glucose release, but whilst this energy is in use, adrenaline output acts to prevent digestion and excretion momentarily, so that all energy response is temporarily reserved for use by muscles. As a manufactured drug, adrenaline helps asthmatics to breathe and is also used by injection to revive heart attack victims.

Once glucose reaches muscles, it requires oxygen to initiate the combustion process that forms carbon dioxide. Only then can energetic muscle movement occur. We expel this carbon dioxide from our lungs as exhaled breath. With each intake of air, we breathe in nitrogen and oxygen primarily, though it is mixed with a little carbon dioxide. Oxygen is taken down into the lungs, where it crosses blood vessel walls to be absorbed into the bloodstream. Here, it combines with glucose at the very end of the digestive process to create life. If muscles are resting or inert, they can manage briefly without oxygen. This is the normal second-by-second assimilation and usage of glucose in our bodies.

Excess sugar is expelled in urine and, most importantly to this book, also used by intestinal yeast/Candida spores as their own energy supply. When yeasts absorb this sugar, wherever it happens, either within intestines or, by analogy, in beer brewing and bread making, it converts to alcohol. This alcohol, through further distillation, becomes antiseptic in quality, and as such, may also be involved in the constant battling between bacteria and yeasts back in the intestines. Antiseptic is a killer of bacteria and alcohol is bacteria-free.

Gases are also produced in the colon as a result of bacterial fermentation and certain vegetables such as onions, cabbage, sprouts, nuts and prunes. One alcohol formed by glucose and yeasts during fermentation is called mannitol; another is methane.

Alcohol - absorption and excretion

Alcohol, formed by the action of yeasts and glucose as well as ingested from alcoholic beverages, is an intense irritant to mucus membranes everywhere in the body. Absorption can begin in the mouth if alcohol is drunk, but when formed from yeast activity in the intestines, it travels across the villi of the intestines into the tiny blood capillaries and then into the bloodstream to travel body-wide.

When it reaches the liver, it is already a highly energised liquid and forces the liver to put it at the head of the queue for energy distribution. This means that good-quality carbohydrates, fats and proteins are made to wait, thereby depriving the body of quality energy and distributing short-action alcoholic energy only. Vitamin absorption is also impaired, which has consequences for enzyme stimulation and causes further digestive interference. (This certainly occurs with far-reaching results in drinkers, but may also be true for people with an already high sugar intake, where excess sugars in alcohol encourage yeasts or Candida in the intestine to overgrow, creating carbon dioxide gas and alcohol. Candidal response to glucose is just that - a response. Candida does not create glucose, it eats it.)

The liver chooses what to do with alcohol. It sends most of it out in the constantly flowing bloodstream to body tissues and muscles for energy, but, when present in quantity, alcohol also acts as an anaesthetic. People who are drunk either do not feel pain at all or feel it at a greatly reduced level. Excess alcohol is also quickly taken up in the kidneys as a poisonous substance for quick excretion in bladder urine; some is excreted in expelled breath, as in the carbon dioxide expulsion process, and some is excreted as sweat. As with the after-effects of ingested alcohol (increased short-term excitement followed by lethargy and sleep), so the chronic sufferer of Candida can describe acute lethargy as one of the symptoms. Drinkers of alcohol are also carriers of above-average yeast activity. This, in men, may not be troublesome, though Candida can be transmitted from seminal fluids in the penis to a receptive female vagina.

Alcohol, when mixed with water (the main component of the bloodstream), can also prove an efficient antiseptic. Pure alcohol is not so efficient, but the mixture of roughly seventy per cent alcohol to thirty per cent water becomes antiseptic. This, in the bloodstream, should therefore act upon bacteria, but in some instances, as with antibiotics, it may leave a yeast overgrowth unaffected. We will discuss this later. It is also interesting to note that pure sugar was used as a wound healer in past centuries. Wounds were heavily layered with sugar or honey and exposed to air - glucose and oxygen. This congealed and formed an alcoholic residue which became antiseptic - anti-bacterial. Again, this will be discussed later.

Within our digestion and absorption processes, lower amounts of alcohol (not those formed by alcoholic drinking) will still travel the same bloodstream-to-tissue routes in continuing cycles, with alcohol deposits occurring body-wide in varying quantities for the purpose of producing energy.

Summary

This chapter has made a reasonable stab at understanding what is a highly complex, interactive chemical process. One component depends upon another component, which influences another and another, and so on. It's almost worse than looking at a genealogical chart of family history - marriages and births expand it all the time until it runs off the sheet of paper and loses all concept of time and personalities. Perhaps we should try to highlight sugar's formation route and function:

Eating- breakdown- absorption- sifting- storage- release into tissues- alcohol and carbon dioxide activity- excretion of carbon dioxide and alcohol in breath or urine.

We are constantly processing and manufacturing sugar in the form of glucose in our digestive system. The system is designed to do this with quality carbohydrates, fats and proteins. It is not designed to do this with extra sugar or alcohol levels from low-quality ingested foodstuffs. By ingesting low-quality, short-lived energy-inducing foods, we over-extend, over-stretch and damage this incredibly delicate chemical balance. A very great deal has been written about this by medical scientists and researchers. Unfortunately, we are not listening; our senses of sight, smell and taste are being bombarded by the marketing of goodies designed to appeal to the sweet-tooth of the twentieth century. Our bodies are naturally complaining.

CHAPTER FOUR

Diabetes

Diabetes costs the USA $132 billion per year of which $91.8 goes in direct medical costs and $40.2 in indirect losses like work, disability and premature death. It is the 6th leading cause of death in the States showing up on death certificates either as an underlying or contributory factor. Diabetics are twice as likely to die as non-diabetics and in the age group 25-44 years there is a 3.6 greater risk of death. It is common in overweight and obese people of both sexes and in all age ranges where food consumption is unrestricted.

Clearly, since diabetics have a sugar problem that can initiate Candida or Thrush, this book needs to give time to the condition and so I have included a small new chapter in this revision. Candida is an additional misery to be dealt with if you are a diabetes sufferer.

What is Diabetes?

Diabetes Mellitus is a long-term, progressive condition in which patients are unable to convert glucose into energy as normal. Insulin, the hormone produced in the beta cells of the pancreas, allows glucose to be used as fuel by the body. In diabetes, there is either a total absence, or insufficient, insulin, due to failure of the beta cells. Without enough insulin, blood glucose concentrations become abnormally high and can lead to serious short or long-term complications.

In non-diabetics, insulin secretion consists of two components: Basal levels, secreted at 1 unit per hour during the night and whilst fasting, and Mealtime levels. Mealtime levels come out 5-10 times above basal levels and are secreted after eating.

There are two types of Diabetes Mellitus simply known as Type 1 and Type 2.

Type 1 is the diagnosis for someone producing little or no insulin because most of their beta cells have been destroyed and can no longer produce insulin at all to regulate glucose. It usually appears in people under forty years of age, often in childhood but actually 15% can start in puberty.

Type 1 can start very quickly with symptoms arriving within a few weeks so many people are unaware until things considerably worsen. Of all diabetic sufferers, Type 1 patients only comprise around 15 % of the total.

Although much research cannot find a sure answer for the beta cells failing to produce insulin, it is felt that viral infections or disease may trigger an auto immune response. Genetics are also thought to play a part.

However if you go into the anti-mercury literature there are other reasons.

Type 2 shows in testing that Beta cells are failing to produce sufficient insulin or even that the body is failing in some way to respond to insulin production. It has a slower onset and symptoms may initially be attributed to just getting old. Awareness is even slower and some systemic damage may have occurred by the time medical help is sought. Type 2 usually appears in people over forty years of age but is common in the obese and is now appearing in fat children whose diet is rich in poor quality foods and whose lifestyle promotes little exercise.

85% of all diabetics have Type 2 and it is increasing in the population at an alarming rate, largely due to fast food outlets, too much bread and pasta, sugar in everything commercial from baked beans to canned drinks, heavier alcohol intake, lack of exercise to burn off the spare glucose and eating much more anyway.

MERCURY INFLUENCE

Insulin is produced in the pancreas. The process of synthesizing insulin requires the formation of sulfur-based bonds between two chains of molecules. Mercury, by interference with and attraction to sulfur-binding sites, can inhibit the production of insulin which, being insufficient to control glucose, then causes glucose levels to rise in the blood like a blocked drain. If individually, insulin in some people is reduced by mercury leakage from teeth fillings or from occupations involving use of mercury or even from eating fish non-stop, then glucose levels may elevate. Diabetes may click in. If there is irregular intake of mercury it would be difficult to diagnose diabetes because of the fluctuation. Mercury latches on to other metal elements in blood and tissue. Manganese, chromium, magnesium and calcium levels may lower causing cramping for instance. Manganese, chromium, Vitamin C and other dietary factors are involved with mercury ingestion, absorption, chelation and ejection. Sulfur is a known mercury- chelating agent.

Mercury vapour and particulate come off dental fillings 24 hours a day, even more with hot food, chewing and acidic alcohol. If fish is eaten a lot there is an enhanced mercury burden. Mercury rises in a thermometer as the temperature rises but it is contained within the glass; nothing contains the vapour rising from the top of a dental filling. It is breathed into the airways and some swallowed with food or drink.

Blood cholesterol levels can be lowered by excessive exercise to a point at which dietary influence fails. How healthy is the gym? Mercury can lower this already low level still further. Safe amalgam removal has been seen to reduce the need for insulin in some patients.

Other risk factors include pregnant women who have birthed a baby weighing more than 8lb8ozs; belonging to South Asian, Hispanic or African descent.

Diabetes symptoms

Victims fit into two categories;

HYPO-GLYCAEMIA

Is where blood sugar levels are dangerously low causing 'events' or sometimes fits. One in six diabetics will at some point have a spell in hospital and most diabetics have at least one hypoglycaemic event a week. 'Hypos' may develop fits, loss of consciousness, coma and even death in severe cases where medical intervention comes too late. Apart from daily treatment, it is essential but difficult to regulate blood sugar levels which can drop during sleep when the patient may not be awake to take instant remedial action.

Hypo-glycaemia is aggravating and frustrating to live with apart from being life-threatening. Despite a pre-meal injection, any delay in eating a meal can interfere with the insulin performance. Symptoms would include sweating, fuzzy vision, faintness, nausea, irritability, confusion, and perhaps loss of consciousness. Anything over this is treated as a medical emergency. Too much exercise in short bursts or long sessions can cause decreased insulin so individuals need to treat their body carefully and know their limits. Such patients wear a MedicAlert bracelet or necklet to alert those either nearby, or medical personnel, to the danger. Symptoms of irritability and confusion can dangerously be legitimately mistaken for being drunk. 'Hypos' may find it a bore but there is more re-assurance if they tell office colleagues, friends and associates that they have this condition. Candida may also be found at a chronic low level.

There are certain risk groups of 'Hypos' where warning symptoms may lessen over time, change or be absent. Those in whom glycaemia is markedly improved; those who develop hypoglycaemia gradually; the elderly; those with a long history of diabetes; those suffering psychiatric illness; those receiving other concurrent medications; all these may experience severe hypoglycaemia with possible loss of consciousness.

Close monitoring, adherence to diet and exercise regimes, not missing meals, stress relief encouraging better insulin sensitivity, watching alcohol consumption and changing the injection area are some of the essential points of which a 'hypo' needs to be aware. Miserably, hypoglycaemic events can also occur from an accidental overdose of insulin and so this condition must be frustrating and difficult to live with.

HYPER-GLYCAEMIA

Is where blood sugar levels are abnormally high causing long-term chronic illnesses because there is insufficient natural insulin present in the bloodstream. Blindness, kidney failure, foot ulceration, erectile dysfunction, heart disease and stroke are some of the main problems. Candida will be an ongoing background problem for many unless sugars are regulated well. Candida loves sugar and thrives on it; most diabetics have a long-term struggle with the additional miseries and symptoms of Candida.

Short term symptoms of sugar overload for a diabetic can include

* dehydration
* blurred vision
* increased levels of skin infection

All advisors helping a diabetic with hyperglycaemia strongly advocate lifestyle changes.

* Eat regular meals
* Eat high fibre foods
* Cut down fat
* Eat more vegetables
* Stop or limit sugary foods and drinks
* Reduce salt consumption
* Reduce weight slowly but surely
* Take regular, gentle exercise
* Stop smoking to reduce heart damage, gangrenous feet and amputation

In both 'hypo' and 'hyper' cases of glycaemia, regulated, daily, personalized doses of insulin are vital. A recent treatment advance, Lantus, manufactured by Aventis Pharma, is a 24-hour insulin therapy used each evening to help patients achieve personal target levels of blood sugar. Any age person can deal with the pre-dosed pen coming in differently measured dosages to be delivered just under the skin not deep into muscle. Lantis comes in vials for injection, cartridge also for injection and the OptiSet pen/plunger for sub-cutaneous pressure. More research is in hand for its suitability with children self-administering and for patients with impaired liver or kidney function. See www.aventis.com and talk to your doctor.

Other tablets and injections can be less reliable and may need to be done more than once a day, nevertheless, they have kept many diabetics alive where once they might have died. Many diabetics have to inject with insulin before mealtimes and sugar levels are usually managed on an individual programme.

Impaired Glucose Intolerance, IgI is a condition approaching diabetes but not yet technically diabetes.An oral glucose tolerance test will show elevated sugar levels and around 16 million people aged between 40 and 70 years old have this condition in America.   It is relieved by reducing sugar, food and alcohol consumption.

Other help abounds these days and this short section linking up sugar levels to Candida and serious illness is of interest to those with or without diabetes. For further help write to: Aventis, 50, Kings Hill Avenue, West Malling, Kent. ME19 4AH. For a list of websites and addresses for diabetes information go into www.google.com on the web and search for yourself.

www.diabetes.niddk.nih.gov/dia/pubs/statistics

is the USA government site but there are plenty more and many useful books in libraries or bookshops.

5 Influence of medicines on Candida upsurge

Antibiotics

If you are reading this book in sequence, you will have already come across historical mentions of anti-sepsis, antiseptics and antibiotics. We are now going to take a detailed look at early and modern kinds of these, some of their names, their action in our bodies, how they are discovered and manufactured and their side-effects.

We pick up the story from Sir Alexander Fleming's accidental discovery in 1928 of a dish of bacteria left exposed to air. After some days, he noticed mould growing on it and that something was now restricting the continuing growth of the bacteria. This mould was Penicillium notatum, and from it he began work on cultivating and observing mould action on bacteria. However, it took years of painstaking work to achieve pure penicillin for trials on humans, and it was only in 1941, when two Oxford scientists, Howard Florey and Ernst Chain, had perfected it, that penicillin was first administered.

Results were immediately impressive and with Fleming, Florey and Chain receiving the Nobel prize in 1945 for their life-saving work, efforts began in the growing pharmaceutical companies to research and manufacture antibiotics. Gonorrhoea, syphilis, gangrene and sepsis from wounds were taking a huge toll of the men in the battle-zones of World War II. Once supplies were dealing adequately with the great wartime demands, home market possibilities opened up.

Life-threatening conditions, such as kidney disease, pneumonia and tuberculosis, began to be successfully treated. These were rife amongst all ages, needing sanitoriums for treatment and recovery, as well as isolation for inhibiting the spread of disease. Antibiotics were, and probably still are, seen as the wonder drug of the twentieth century and have played an enormous part in population explosions. Where once the survival of the fittest controlled populations modern medicine has now interfered and saved millions of lives through infection control. The same can be said of improved public and personal hygiene, purer water, hospital treatments and medical advances. The world has welcomed it all but our natural resources are in decline and eventually like many fish and water stocks much will be used up.

MORE RECENT DEVELOPMENTS

Antibiotics and their miraculous life-saving properties became a mainstay of health. Only in the 1990s, with escalating State Healthcare costs and doubts about irresponsible prescribing, have attempts been made to do without them unless really necessary. These doubts include:

- bacterial resistance to older forms of antibiotics because of the ability of bacteria to mutate or change their genetic structures and avoid being killed off. Some have proved to be highly efficient at repelling attempts to eradicate them, and indeed hospital infection rates are rising all the time;
- risk to the immune system, which we shall deal with later on, meaning that the natural way in which immunity repels bacterial invasion or upsurge has been compromised or damaged.

I was born in 1941 and was a sickly child. From the age of four until eleven, my life was made miserable by allergies, bronchitis, asthma and several episodes of resultant pneumonia. Nothing at that time helped multi-allergies, which included moulds, dust, feathers, hay, grass, cereals, dogs, cats, house-dust mite, pollens and a great array of foodstuffs, fumes and additives. I would have clearly died before reaching puberty had it not been for M&B.

M&B stood for May and Baker, a pharmaceutical firm, researching and marketing early penicillin tablets. At regular intervals, probably every eight to ten weeks, the doctor would have to be called out, despite my mother's attempts to ease my breathing difficulties by upturning steaming kettles of Friars Balsam. The two white M&B tablets, as we knew them, were used to save and prolong my young life.

Even though an osteopath manipulating my ribs and spine caused a hundred per cent cessation of the bronchitis and asthma in 1953, I was left with terrible allergic rhinitis which regularly caused ear and sinus infections. These, too, required M&B tablets, until they were overtaken by other pharmaceutical developments. I have fallen victim to more than my fair share of coughs and colds, often requiring penicillin or its advancing derivatives for severe infections. We now know that vapourising mercury from many teeth fillings begun aged 4 and a half have been responsible for all this and ruining the mucosal lining of my sinuses.

I married at the age of twenty-four, and the story of my seven years on antibiotics for cystitis is well documented in chapter 1. Urinary infections can scar the kidneys, and kidney disease was the biggest killer of women until antibiotics arrived. In short, I am an antibiotic child of the twentieth century. Death would have overtaken me at almost any time from natural progression of severe infections in my lungs or kidneys. But I was also born at the time of huge, life-saving advances in medicine. There have been many pleasures and plans, but, equally, the restriction caused by ill-health has been frustrating. There are many others like me.

Infections are not always life-threatening, fearful experiences. We recover and live; what is of great concern to all of us is the effect of this love affair with anti-bacterial drugs. Have we paved the way for some enormous, futuristic plague? Some people would quietly say that this might be so, that indeed we may be experiencing the opening gambits of yeast takeovers. Their upsurges are increasingly frequent, and we would do well to look more closely at this so-called wonder drug which has proved to be one of the top triggers of yeast epidemics.

HOW ARE ANTIBIOTICS MANUFACTURED?

Early growths of antibiotic substances in laboratories were made on small culture dishes, but then went on to be manufactured in row upon row of milk bottles slanted on shelves to achieve maximum aeration. In England, improving production was difficult because of bombing raids in the 1940s, so the American pharmaceutical firm Pfizer, based in Brooklyn, after much discussion and experimenting on purifying penicillin, began vat-style production. Each fermentation tank at the factory was able to produce 10,000 gallons of crude antibiotic liquid, or broth as they called it. By 1943, emphasis on producing penicillin and additional strains was the second highest government production programme next to the race to manufacture the atomic bomb.

The whole science is dependent upon one main observation, which says that microbes 'compete' with each other and therefore have an ability to attack and invade, as well as to defend and resist. As bacterial and microbiological studies took off, so were experimental 'coincidences' inhibiting bacterial growth discovered.

Whilst World War II undoubtedly brought horror and destruction, it can also be argued that it was a great trigger in encouraging collaboration between medical and pharmaceutical bodies. This collaboration meant that large-scale factories and purification systems were needed worldwide to service increasing demand for penicillins, streptomycins, sulphonamides, tetracyclines, cephalosporins and dozens more. Continuous discoveries both in drugs, bacteria and yeasts meant that by the mid-1990s, over 6,000 antibiotics had been licensed. Anti-fungal medications would soon follow.

Many early drug companies soon began to market antibiotics as the wonder drug and life-saver. Production escalated everywhere, often in response to geographical locations able to provide and sustain constant supplies of the basic, raw plant life needed to fill huge fermentation tanks with nutrients, liquids and fermenting properties from which the processed antibiotic could emerge. Early penicillin was administered by injection, but with the discovery in 1957 of the first semi-synthetic antibiotic, called Methicillin, derived from penicillins, administration by mouth as tablets became commonplace rather than occasional.

Modern antibiotics are still mostly based on plant or vegetation mould or fungal fermentation. The moulds can also be drawn from soils where organisms called actinomycetes are able to produce antibacterial actions. Antibiotics act on infection sites in differing ways:

- bacteriostatic: inhibits powers of growth in the infection bacterium by interfering with its digestive system, so weakening its ability to multiply. Some other bacteriostatic antibiotics stop formation of the **cell** structure of the infection bacterium. Other actions can include interfering with cell membrane, enzyme production and genetic malfunction;
- bactericidal: kills infection bacteria totally.

BACTERIAL RESISTANCE TO ANTIBIOTICS

Having evolved since the planet was first formed, it is obvious that bacteria have vast resources for survival. Genetic, mutational and synthesised reactions to invasion, attack and growth inhibition are not new skills. Survival spirit within micro-organisms appears infinite. We should be in awe of these unseen predators who continue to plague us, no matter what we fling at them. This resistance by bacteria to other bacterial strains and to our human efforts has been noted and documented since the early penicillin laboratory discoveries, but sixty years on, it is now far more advanced.

In 1940, Ernst Chain and Edward Abraham showed that E. Coli, the commonest intestinal group of infection-causing bacteria, had produced an enzyme named penicillinase. This clever enzyme, now known as a lactamase, can help many kinds of bacteria to stay alive in spite of penicillin treatment. As this enzyme action was researched on other bacteria, it was found to be present in many strains, effectively throwing a spanner into the new-found works.

Penicillin in its first forms began to look far less formidable as an anti-bacterial agent, and bacterial engineering had to begin.

Additives to counteract lactamase were sought, and new antibiotics were constantly developed to fight bacterial ability to save itself. Penicillinase has been found in Egyptian mummies, whose ancient secrets have opened up under modern microbiology. This cunning, cell-saving enzyme did not evolve in answer to modern antibiotics, but has been genetically present in humans since life began.

For the purpose of prescribing antibiotics, bacteria are classified as one of the following:

- resistant to (meaning that the bacteria refuse to die in the face of the antibiotic therapy on test culture);
- sensitive to (meaning that the bacteria have not found a way to fight off or survive the antibiotic therapy. This antibiotic will then be chosen to treat the patient.).

After fifty years, waging war on such resistance is still a full-time job for scientists. It is said that 'every course of antibiotics gives bacteria the chance to develop resistance', and that early, indiscriminate use has devalued the worth of the wonder drug. Despite this, sixty per cent of doctors in America still prescribe antibiotics for minor viruses and infections. In developing countries, bacterial resistance is escalating because prescription controls do not exist. Africa, Asia and the Middle East all have these drugs for sale in pharmacies without prescription.

Tuberculosis is now on the increase in the United Kingdom, where it was thought to have been eradicated in the 1970s by antibiotics and vaccines. It has been re-introduced by foreign travel, street spitting and warmer air. Aeroplanes, trains, boats and cars act like a laboratory culture dish with thriving bacteria enclosed in warmth on moist clothing and skin debris. Transmission by contact or breath is easy. The intermingling of cultures; the lack, in many countries of hygiene; bacterial resistance to drugs or misuse of drugs; these are not only features in rising reports of tuberculosis, but also of many other infections.

Hospitals, once places of superb levels of cleanliness and healing, are now proving to be enlarged culture plates. Hospital bedding, clothing, floors, walls and instruments are all receiving resistant strains of bacteria from sick patients. Large wards, warmth, sickly people, staff and visitor movements spread infection rapidly.

Antibiotic resistance is reported all over the world. Gentamicin, for instance, which is in very common use, particularly for staphylococcus groups of bacteria, can be virtually useless against sixty per cent of these bacteria in the USA and thirty-seven per cent in Zaire, both places where indiscriminate use has been allowed.

In veterinary practice, antibiotics are given regularly. Thirty-five per cent of pigs and ten per cent of chickens in American food production facilities are fed antibiotics randomly. Drug companies in the USA are insistent that antibiotic resistance has not increased, but since antibiotics are excreted in urine as well as assimilated in the bloodstream of such animals, both their flesh and their excrement waste must contain antibiotics. In the food chain, this is passed on for human consumption.

Vegetable and salad production for en masse supplies into supermarkets are heavily sprayed. Soil is carefully prepared for maximum productivity by pesticides and antiseptic solutions. We eat them along with the food! Their action is anti-bacterial, anti-fungal and destroys the balance of micro-organisms. From every conceivable direction meat, greens, fruits, cereals, drugs, travel, air, excrement, we now find human beings bombarded with antibiotics. We are becoming more susceptible to coughs, colds and bacterial infections, as well as having a predisposition to yeast/ Candida infestations. The fight for balance, internally and externally, is becoming increasingly difficult; we must take antibiotic therapy as a serious, last option, not a quick fix.

PHARMACEUTICAL RESPONSE

The genetic engineering of antibiotic ingredients is opening up the manufacture of new derivatives from known antibiotic groups, and enzyme changes, too, have caused excitement. Gyrase, an enzyme which helps bacteria to reproduce, has now been inhibited by chemical engineering, and this has resulted in a new group of antibiotic compounds called quinolones. Norfloxacin, enoxacin and ciprofloxacin can also be used where more common antibiotics are now failing. Enzyme-inhibiting factors are now at the forefront of new antibiotic research, and researchers hold out much hope for this line of enquiry.

Vaccination against bacterial infection is also under investigation in many research centres, but all vaccines contain ingredients harmful to human health such as Thimerosal- a preservative containing mercury. Vaccines also contain large numbers of animal viruses indicated in vaccine-induced illnesses. But there is now another interesting avenue of anti-bacterial work being undertaken. When discussion of terminology for drugs combating bacterial infection and sepsis took place in the late 1930s, settling finally for 'antibiotic', not everyone in research was happy about it.

Selman Waksman in the USA held the day, but the construction is interesting: 'anti' means 'against', biotic' means 'life', which, at first glance, seems to imply that the drug is 'against life'. It certainly works against the lives of the bacteria which cause infection but, quickly said, it has the deeper meaning 'against human interest'.

The opposite word, 'probiotic' ('pro' meaning 'for'), can be more constructive from the patient's viewpoint. A probiotic is a supporter of life. This opens a whole new range of drug possibilities and emphasis.

Probiotics

The action of antibiotics is either to inhibit enzyme activity or to kill outright those major groups of bacteria in air, water or soil which invade, infect or inhabit the human body. Broad spectrum antibiotics affect bacteria other than those specifically causing the trouble and after a five-seven-ten-day course or longer of antibiotics, the flora of the intestines is greatly affected. With large numbers of bacteria being killed off, the balance is disturbed between bacteria and yeasts. Candida, particularly, is no longer held in check and upsurges, since it faces no opposing bacterial forces with any strength left.

Probiotic bacteria have two functions: they aid digestion processes, in particular helping the intestines to achieve a healthy peristalsis (passing of food particles and chyme towards the bowel), so that less time is taken in excreting waste. This helps regulate bacterial build-up and controls toxins; and they actively discourage the reproduction of toxinous bacteria like coliforms, streptococcus and others. Since both toxic and probiotic bacteria need their own territory, they too, fight for their own survival like yeasts versus bacteria.

We already know from chapter 2 that the stomach is so acidic that few known bacteria survive in it, and we also know that the duodenum and jejunum have very little bacterial or yeast activity. We know that great colonies of bacteria and yeasts thrive from the small intestine onwards. We also know that yeasts, apart from needing moisture and glucose, also prefer a mild acidic or alkaline environment. If there is sufficient acidity in the small intestine, yeasts will be inhibited. Yet this factor of acidity within each of us varies. Blood is slightly alkaline anyway, but if the small and large intestines are suffering from regularly ingested foodstuffs inclining the system towards alkalinity, then yeasts clearly thrive.

Maintaining the acid-alkaline balance is therefore a good objective. We certainly can't attain the gastric acidity of the stomach, but we can try to encourage intestinal bacteria which produce acidity. These are:

Lactobacillus
This group includes acidophilus, kefir, bulgaricus, plantarum, casei, brevis, salivarius, delbrueckii, jugurti and thermophilus. All these help produce lactic acid, most particularly from carbohydrate foodstuffs (potatoes, rice, pasta, etc.). Some are found in certain yoghurts and some cheeses, but these are not always

helpful, since fungi are added for taste and fermentation and carbohydrates convert eventually into glucose. Some are long-term inhabitants of the intestines, but some are not, being eaten and excreted within the digestive time-spans.

Bifidobacteria

The three major bifidobacteria (bifidum, infantis and longum) form a dominant colony in the intestines but they can be overtaken by toxinous bacteria in sickness, by stressed immune responses, under antibiotic therapy, in alkalinity and poor diet. Ageing causes them to decline.

Their action is one of acid level maintenance by formation and production of acetic acid and lactic acid. Many of the toxinous bacteria do not thrive well in acid mediums. By stimulating acid production in the intestines, a level of balance may be maintained.

Streptococci

Some of these, which either pass through or normally inhabit the intestines, can be helpful because they produce the enzyme lactase which helps break down sugars in milk and dairy products. They can also produce lactic acid, but, because they also count as infection bacteria, they are less useful in encouraging a healthy environment.

Because we are so finely balanced and affected by external forces of diet, illness, climate, clothing, stress, work, sex, family, drugs, alcohol and a host of lifestyle affectations, it is impossible to standardise our intestinal environment. Clearly, taking excessive probiotics would equally create an imbalance of intestinal bacteria and yeasts. Later on I shall be giving guidelines for daily probiotic influence and also probiotic response therapy for Candida upsurges.

BACTERIAL INTERACTION

If bacteria all have common controlling and inhibiting abilities, how do they achieve this? It is an inspirational inter-dependence! For example, bifidobacteria being anaerobes, require an absence of oxygen to thrive, so they depend upon the presence and activity of oxygen-loving bacteria. Aerobes such as coliforms, staphs, streps, klebsiella, proteus and pseudomonas consume oxygen and it is usually the presence of aerobes in infection sites which require antibiotic therapy. Antibiotics, in turn, help promote Candidal growth, completing the degeneration of organism balance.

Probiotic replacement therapy could now be useful. The action of probiotics is friendly. It is kindly, encouraging and replacing rather than inhibiting or destructive. It, too, because of replenishment and maintenance, is life-saving. Attention to healthy digestion means less likelihood of infection, though major diseases, such as tuberculosis, pneumonia, venereal disease and kidney disease, would require antibiotic administration. Each one of us must look after our own health through proper use of public and personal hygiene, environmental epidemic control, correct intake of minerals and vitamins, and try to minimise our need for antibiotics.

The use of probiotics is the result of recent research and findings. It is not always accepted by some of those scientists who have been at the forefront of medical and pharmaceutical developments. Nevertheless, probiotic use is now favoured when possible, by the public. Orion Truss, Leon Chaitow, William Crook and other researchers have begun to prod at the establishment. It is obvious to everyone that friendly organisms, such as lactobacillus and bifidobacteria, exist; it is the role of these organisms that is now under research and rightly so. We do not only want knowledge of unfriendly, life-threatening bacteria. There needs to be a balance in research, just as there needs to be intestinal balance of bacteria and yeasts.

Dental Amalgams relating to Candida levels

At the same time as my attacks of bronchitis and pneumonia ceased in 1953, my first heavy session of dental treatment began. It was dreadful. My dentist, a frequent lunchtime drinker, was not disposed to use injections to dull pain, and, with a sensitive mouth, the black chair and the drilling into my double teeth was complete torture. I went under great duress, and not until there remained no choice but to treat the toothache. Although I had made the usual ineffective childhood efforts to clean my teeth, by the age of eleven, they were in dire need of treatment. Sickly in bed for so long, cleaning was often missed and sweets, although limited, were reasonably regular as little treats in this deprived lifestyle.

By the age of twelve, I had a quarter of my teeth filled with varying amounts of metal amalgams, mercury always being dominant like an egg binds cake together, except that mercury constitutes 60%. Over the years, more amalgam was added, including four double teeth root-canaled between 1986 and 1987. In 1987, I had two porcelain crowns and two gold crowns inserted so only eight front teeth remained without any dental treatment. In 1987, I went down with so-called ME/Chronic Fatigue Syndrome. It was actually a toxic response to the mercury and gold dental work at that time.

I am not uncommon as a modern dental patient. Until the arrival of dental anaesthesia, most people avoided the dentist's chair because of pain. Extraction was the recognised remedy for bad teeth, and once full sets of dentures were available, particularly on the emergent National Health Service in the late 1940s, many people endured the new injections and removal of all their teeth rather than suffer. This was usually done over a few weeks and new dentures were then provided.

Dentistry grew apace of new findings, new research, new drilling techniques and new anaesthetics, whether local injections, gas and air, or intravenous injections. This would have been fine but for two things:

- the increase of sugar in a vast array of foodstuffs, especially those aimed at babies and children. Sugar consumption over the centuries has risen along with the figures for tooth decay,
- the increase of sugars and refined flours in the daily diet.

Sugary foods and drinks have a greater ability to adhere to tooth enamel. Before food refinement in factories, most people, except the wealthiest, could not afford these more expensive foodstuffs. Food was bulkier, more fibrous and husky, all of which took time to chew. The size of the food particles remaining in tooth crevices was larger than those today; these particles could not get wedged in for hours at a time to initiate decay, nor were they so sugary or sticky. Even so, honey, alcohol and failure to clean led to rapid dental decay and diseased teeth which were either pulled or simply fell out.

Dentists these days recommend cleaning teeth after each meal, and we are told to use floss or tiny brushes to clean out the cracks. This is to prevent today's diet of minute particles adhering to enamel in inaccessible cracks.

MERCURY AMALGAM

Because of anaesthetics and improved dental techniques, most people have amalgam fillings. But before 1820, teeth were either pulled or filled with gold if you could afford it. To overcome the costs of gold fillings, persuade patients to put money into dental pockets and to preserve a tooth structure, amalgam 'plugs' were made up of zinc, copper, tin and silver. These were held together with liquid mercury. This practice began in England in 1819 with a dentist called Mr Bell, and by the late 1820s, was in use throughout Europe and the USA.

By 1830, dentists and doctors were debating whether it was wise to put mercury, a known poison and antiseptic, into people's mouths. By 1840, the National Association of Dental Surgeons in the USA had banned its use for teeth fillings because it was known to be so dangerous. However, the cost of mercury fillings was not only kind to patients, but also to dental pockets since more patients came for the cheaper treatments.

As a result, amalgam continued to be used elsewhere. Eventually the American Dental Surgeons Association failed and folded because its membership declined as unlicensed 'quacks' attracted the public away with cheaper mercury fillings. It gave in after fifteen years, safeguarded its pockets and re-invented the mercury filling!

Today, both the modern British and American Dental Associations ignore the known poisonous and antiseptic nature of mercury in favour of the cheapness of mercury amalgams. Modern opposition is vociferous; some manufacturers of mercury amalgam are sensing future litigation and are phasing out production. The World Health Organisation has stated its opposition to amalgams, and several countries in Europe have placed restriction and banning orders on it.

The game is up for dentists, despite 170 years of largely successful efforts to fool themselves, as well as patients by covering up systemic poisoning from inhalation of mercury vapour and ingestion of particulate.

Safe removal of mercury amalgams has to be carried out using the strictest precautions against mercury vapour inhalation or ingestion; if precautions are not taken, greater risk of toxicity is present, with detrimental effects on the health of both dentist and patient. Minimally, these precautions should be using a rubber dam to isolate the quadrant or tooth being treated, high-speed drill, oxygen mask, head coverings, eye coverings, ten days of strong mins/vits to help protect the immune system, two charcoal tablets taken minutes before treatment commences. All dental staff should be well covered, surgery regularly 'swept' and no mercury residue should be put down toilets.

ACTION OF MERCURY

In chapter 1, I made passing mention of early attempts to fight infections prior to antisepsis and later antibiotics. One of these early attempts found that minute quantities of mercury were useful as an antiseptic in combating infection. Mercury is an antiseptic; it has been and still is used as an antiseptic in hundreds of pharmaceutical and industrial products, and, as such, it has powers to inhibit bacterial activity.

It follows that, when you inhibit bacteria, yeasts surge into the territory now available. Mercury is not taken like a course of antibiotics, but as a filling in the mouth, it provides a 24-hour release for the duration of the filling. As vapour and droplets are breathed or swallowed, there is a regular drip-feed of it into the bloodstream via intestinal villi and lung capillaries. Mercury lodges within major organs and can be deposited in tissue and bone all over the body, as proven by recent research.

As this antiseptic drips and gathers around the body, it disturbs not only bacteria and yeast levels, it affects hormone balance. Hormones, particularly insulin, affect blood sugar and glucose levels. These may become less stable, encouraging, with more glucose, the nutritional requirements for Candida.

Mercury can also cause zinc deficiency, which interferes with enzyme production in the pancreas, resulting in higher levels of body alcohol. Of course, Candida depends upon glucose and alcohol for nutrition. And whilst having antiseptic qualities, mercury is highly toxic in prolonged or heavy accidental doses. Many people have allergies to metals, which show up as rashes caused by jewellery. Nickel in jewellery or dental materials can badly affect some people.

SUMMARY

Mercury amalgams affect hormones, sugar control and levels, allergic reactions, bacteria/yeast balance, immunity responses, Candida or yeast infections. It has been called the toxic time-bomb, and is in use in an incredible number of products, including throat lozenges, herbicides, insecticides, industrial processes, spermicidal creams/gels, fabric softeners, jewellery, chlorine production, gardening chemicals, tile grout, photographic solutions, vaginal medications, haemorrhoidal ointments and suppositories, ear/nose/ throat medications, acne medication, bleaches, psoriasis creams, anti-fungal preparations and many antiseptics used in the home. With all of these in regular use, having fillings in our mouths made from mercury amalgams seems to be the final straw.

Following amalgam and cap removal under stringent dental and nutritional conditions, my own nine years bedbound with so-called ME/CFS and including continuous Candida, ended within three months. Mercury increases its toxicity fourfold when gold is added.

Finally, those people who appear to be unaffected by their fillings may not yet have reached their personal threshold of poisoning, this may be instantaneous after dental treatment or it may build slowly and show as strokes in later life. More information is available from PAMA (Patients Against Mercury Amalgams) on www.angela.kilmartin.dial.pipex.com There is a 236 page Compilation of articles, science, letters from sufferers, safe removal, chelation and much more information available.

Such responses to a very commonly used source of a toxic, antiseptic, allergenic substance may well be responsible for lowered resistance and Candidal susceptibility.

Mercury toxicity is responsible for a great many other health problems, but they are not in the remit of this book, except to say that immune system distress in any illness will decrease well-being and allow yeasts either to upsurge or remain as strengthened colonies.

Steroids influencing immune and Candidal response

Steroids are either natural drugs obtained from gland secretions in animals or they are synthetically manufactured to simulate the same function as those animal secretions. They basically comprise hormones, which are then used to inhibit or activate chemical actions which may be malfunctioning and causing ill-health.

CORTISCOSTEROIDS

In 1950, three scientists called Kendall, Richotein and Hench shared a Nobel prize for their discovery that cortiscosteroids, from the cortex of the adrenal glands behind the kidneys, could be life-saving. These drugs help to decrease the effects of shock in the short term and to control inflammation, such as in severe asthma or allergy response. From those early uses, wide ranges of illnesses have now been found to improve symptomatically, that is, the illness itself remains but its worst effects are eased.

Research on steroid drug formulas has changed them greatly over the years, enabling wider use in creams, sprays, inhalers, capsules and tablets for asthma control, rheumatic inflammation, skin irritation, arthritis and lung diseases, amongst others. Unfortunately, steroids also have potentially dangerous side-effects which necessitate careful and regular monitoring by a doctor. These side effects may include:

- Oedema: water retention, especially in feet, legs, hips, back, pelvis and face due to sodium and water retention rather than control and excretion;
- Osteoporosis
- Degenerative arthritis
- Blood vessel weakness
- Spinal degeneration
- Digestive interference: carbohydrates fail to be digested and development of diabetes can arise. Sugar and alcohol levels become too high;
- Peptic ulcers: due to chemical changes in gastric mucus protecting the stomach membrane;
- Sex hormone disturbance: leading to menstrual changes.

Steroid therapy mimics the natural responses of the adrenal cortex, and this has to be re-trained to return to its full function before the course of steroid treatment is concluded. A gradual decrease of the drug is vital.

Cortiscosteroids comprise three sections: glucocorticoids, mineral corticoids and sex hormones.

Cortiscosteroids

Natural	Synthetic
cortisone	prednisone
hydrocortisone	prednisolone
aldosterone	methyprednisolone
cortiscosterone	triamcinolone
deoxycortone	dexamethasone
	betamethasone
	fludrocortisone

As far as Candida is concerned, any disturbance to sugar control is helpful to yeast growth since its chief nutrient for growth is glucose, or glucose then reduced to alcohol. Thus a course of cortiscosteroids, together with the initial illness, doubly reduces immune system strength encouraging Candida upsurge.

SEX HORMONES

These are steroids, too. They occur naturally in both men and women.

In Men

Testosterone is an androgen (male) hormone secreted from cells in the testes. Its effects are to promote mature sexual growth and create spermatozoa. It also stimulates bone growth and strength. Other androgen hormones are excreted by the adrenal cortex, but are not so potent as those from the testes.

Androgen replacement therapy is useful for any normal secretion disturbances, for advanced osteoporosis, acute renal failure, general wasting diseases and some types of female breast cancers. Again, adverse effects dictate a need for careful medical supervision.

Androgens are all synthetic, and the most common are:

methyltestosterone	nandrolone
fluoxmesterone	methandienone
norethandrolone	stanozol

All have adverse effects and are not recommended long term.

In Women

There are two main types of sex hormone in women: oestrogen and progestogen.

Oestrogen comprises oestrone, oestradiol and oestriol, all of which are natural steroids secreted by the ovaries, placenta and the adrenal cortex. The male testes also secrete some oestrogen. Females also secrete progesterone.

Oestrogens help create breasts, maintain the epithelium (lining) of the uterus, create the vulval opening of the developing female foetus, and oversee the general femininity of the female body. Oestrogens are:

Natural	Synthetic
oestrone	stilboestrol (non-steroid)
oestriol	dinoestrol
oestradiol	ethinyloestradiol
	hexoestrol
	methallenoestril
	chlorotrianisene
	mestranol

All of the oestrogen-based hormones can be helpful as prescription medications. They may inhibit breast milk, help menstrual disorders like pre-menstrual tension or Amenorrhoea, decrease some cancers of the breast or prostate gland (in men), induce an abortion or, conversely, improve fertility. They are useful in hormone replacement therapy and in contraceptives.

In progestogens, the natural steroid is known as progesterone and has several functions in the female menstrual cycle: it prepares the uterus for reception of the monthly egg from the ovaries, it can prevent ovulation and calm down the muscles which make the uterus contract and it helps in breast development. Progestogens are:

Natural	Synthetic
progesterone	
ethisterone	
norethisterone	
lynoestrenol	(derivative)
norethynodrel	(derivative)
norethisterone	(derivative)
ethynodiol	(derivative)
norgestrel	(derivative)
hydroxyprogesterone	(derivative)

These are only a few of the progestogens available and experiments are constantly being carried out to find better-tolerated combinations.

In short, oestrogens and progestogens perform natural and synthetic hormone functions. Oral contraceptives and hormone replacement therapies abound now and are derived from differing balances of oestrogens and progestogens. They can produce different side-effects in individual women; rather than give up, women should monitor, record and report their difficulties to their doctor or gynaecologist. The treatment can then be modified as necessary.

As far as Candida is concerned, hormones can, depending again on individual tolerance, immune system response, blood sugar levels, efficient digestion and so on, impair glucose tolerance and raise sugar levels. Fluid may be retained, leaving the kidneys unable to excrete excess glucose and allowing it to remain in circulation. Experimentation and monitoring are recommended. Additionally, the monthly secretion of progesterone to activate bleeding changes vaginal levels of acidity to alkalinity. This is responsible for pre-menstrual vaginal Candida. The alkalinity continues during the bleeding week and a little after to keep an alkaline vagina until oestrogen once again acts alone.

ADRENALINE AND OTHER AMINES

Adrenaline is secreted by the adrenal medulla section of the adrenal glands which lie above and behind the kidneys. We already know that it is useful in emergency breathing situations as a broncho-dilator (enlarging bronchial tubes for increased air flow); adrenaline can also decrease bleeding from an operation or wound, assist anaesthetic action and aid slow absorption of different drugs. Adrenaline and other amines are alkaline.

- noradrenaline: helps in blood circulation and blood pressure;
- dopamine: helps in processes for reducing constriction of arteries which carry blood away from the heart. It helps reduce high blood pressure;
- ephedrine: helps adrenaline and noradrenaline to work to greater effect. It stimulates the central nervous system and has a dilating effect on bronchial tubes, easing asthma, bronchitis and other breathing difficulties. In sinusitis, it decongests stuffed-up or runny noses. It is alkaline and a synthesised steroid;
- amphetamine: is a temporary stimulant, first used to relieve nasal congestion, but now classed as an addictive drug;
- tyramine: helps release noradrenaline and can cause hypertension;
- salbutamol: regulates heartbeat and pulse.

BETA BLOCKERS

There are several varieties of these drugs which primarily stabilise membranes and inhibit secretions which would irritate and inflame local or wider membranes. They, too, are steroids which can prompt yeast upsurge. As there are new drug combinations appearing all the time, you should check all ingredients listed on the leaflets or packaging when starting a new medicine. If in doubt, consult your doctor or pharmacist. Beta blockers are:

acebutol	pindolol
alprenolol	practolol
atenol	propranolol
metoprolol	sotalol
oxprenolol	timolol

LISTS OF COMMON MEDICATIONS

• These are some of the commonly used asthma and allergy medications containing steroids and new compounds which are capable of causing immune suppression, raising alkalinity and impairing sugar/glucose absorption to some degree:

Aerobec, Aerocrom, Aerolin, Alomide, Alphaderm, Alphodith, Alphosyl HC, Alupent, Beckloforte, Beconase, Becotide, Berotec, Betnovate, Bricanyl, Canesten Hydrocortisone, Chioromycetin, Hydrocortisone, Choledyl, Clarityn Daneral S.A., Dermovate, Dexa Rhinaspray, Dimotane, Diprosalic, Diprosone, Dithrocream, Duovent, Efcortelan cream, Elocon, Ephedrine drops, Eumovate, Eurax Hydrocortisone, Exirel, Flixonase, Flixotide, Franol, Galpseud, Gentisone Hydrocortisone, Hismanal, Hydrocal, Hydrocortisyl, Intal, Lasma Locoid Hydrocortisone, Medihaler, Medrone, Metosyn FapG, Modrasone, Neo-Cortef, Nerisone, Otomize, Otosporin, Periactin, Phenergan, Piriton, Prednesol, Preferid, Primalan, Pro-Actidil, Proctofoam HC, Proctosedyl, Propaderm, Pro-vent, Pulmadil, Pulmicort, Quinocort, Quinoderm HC, Rhinocort, Rinatec, Rhinolast, Rynacrom, Salbulin, Scheriproct, Semprex, Serevent, Sofrade, Sudafed, Sudocream, Synalar, Tarcortin, Theo-Dur, Thephorin, Timodine, Topilar, Triludan, Terfenadine, Ultraproct, Ultradil, Uniphyllin, Ventide, Ventolin, Xyloproct.

• These are some of the commonly used hypertensive, vasodilating, anticoagulant drugs, all of which are capable, to varying degrees, of causing yeast upsurge by digestion interference, hormone disturbance and immune system damage; many have an alkaline base:

Accupro, Accuretric Adizem, Aldactide, Apresoline, Arelix, BetaAdalat, Betaloc, Blocadren, Calcilat, Carace, Cardinol, Catapres, Celectol, Co-Betaloc, Decaserpyl,

Declinax, Diurexan, Emcor, Esidrex, Geangin, Hydromet, Hydrosaluric, Hygroton, Hytrin, Inderal, Inderetic, Inderex, Innovace, Ismelin, Kaispare, Kalten, Kerlone, Lasipressin, Lopresor, Lopresoretic, Metenix, Mudocren, Navispare, Nifensar, Suluric, Secadrex, Sectral, Slow-Trasicor, Tenif, Teneroet, Tenoret, Tenormin, Tildiem, Totamol, Trasicot, Trasidex, Tritace, Univer, Vascace, Viskaldix, Visken, Zestoretic, Zestril.

- These are some of the commonly used compounds for depression, anxiety, sleeplessness and decongesting stuffy sinuses:

Amytal, Beta-Prograne, Buspar, chiordiazepoxide, diazepam, Inderal, lorazepam, lormetazepam, nitrazepam, Noctec, Nytol, oxazepam, Oxypertine, Phenergan, Sominex, Stemetil, Soneryl, temazepam, Trancopal, Welidorm, Zimovane.

- Antacids for gastric upsets are of an alkaline nature. Many people are puzzled when, having taken an antacid for stomach indigestion, there is an increase in pain and wind. For these people, peppermint is probably better. Candida enjoys alkalinity, so antacids should be avoided including:

Calcium Carbonate, Bicarbonate of Soda, Algicon, Pyrogastrone.

Insulin

Other, non-sexual hormones play very important roles in glucose formation and absorption. If the metabolic structure or genetic disposition inclines towards certain health difficulties, then replacements of missing or low levels of important components would be likely to reduce or allay the symptoms. Such a case is pancreatic metabolism. If insulin secretion is too low, then blood sugar will accumulate to cause diabetes. Regulation both by insulin treatment given in regular injections and by controlled sugar intake is a daily struggle. Often this careful regulation can be thrown by other factors in daily life, and diabetes requires great patience and perseverance.

Apart from insulin injections and newly available tablets, there are other kinds of drugs which act in a way that perhaps mimics insulin. They are: Tolbutamide, Chlorpropamide, Tolazamide, Acetohexamide and Glibenclamide, which all stimulate pancreatic cells to produce insulin, thereby encouraging sugar storage in the liver. These also appear to help other areas of sugar absorption within the digestive system, so that less reliance is placed upon pancreatic insulin. They can occasionally have side-effects, such as overproduction of lactic acid leading to lactic acidosis, but this is very rare. Certain illnesses involving the kidneys, liver, lungs, heart and blood vessels may also prevent their use. A second sugar-controlling group of drugs includes Phenformin and Metformin.

An innovative type of insulin called Lantus, insulin glargine, will help some 600,000 UK diabetics live more normal lives. It works by a controlled injection from a pen-type device just under the skin. Lantus is easier for teenagers and older people to use since it does not involve a deeper injection into muscle. Ask the doctor about it or write to Aventis Ltd., Aventis House, 50, King's Hill Avenue, West Malling, Kent. ME19 4AH. www.aventis.com

Anaesthetics

There are many different anaesthetics available these days, serving a variety of purposes pertinent to specific operations, patient's needs and swifter recovery. Dental anaesthetics have greatly changed, not only in their pharmacological make-up, but also in better knowledge of just where to inject for the greatest pain relief. It can take several weeks to recover from any anaesthetic; it's not simply a matter of feeling better the next day because spin-offs around the body's metabolism can take far longer to re-balance. Resulting depression and individual responses to digestion, mind, sensory functions, movement and energy may be expected. All of these affect those vital areas of Candida control such as alkalinity, glucose and immune system defence. The following anaesthetics are examples:

Lignocaine, Chinchocaine, antihistamines, cocaine, ethylchloride, alcohol procainamide, adrenaline, Procaine, Prilocaine, Bupivacaine, Amethocaine, Benzocaine.

Chemotherapy and Radiotherapy

These words tend to apply to treatments for cancers of all sorts and at any site in the body. Improved drugs and drips minimising nauseous side-effects are constantly being introduced. Radium treatments are also progressing and help to improve patient response, shorter treatment times and out-patient facilities.

Despite all this, Candidal upsurge may result from treatments which suppress or kill not just the cancerous areas, but also fringe sites. Expect to feel less energetic from the treatments as well as the cancer itself. This combination of treatment and illness undoubtedly affects immune system and defence mechanisms causing them distress and allowing opportunistic Candidal upsurge for some time.

There are now several wonderful cancer books available for patients. They offer common sense approaches and innovative ideas on causes of cancer and remedies other than, or adjunctive, to surgery. Look for Dr. Hulda Clark's "The Cure for all cancers" and Ron Gdanski's "Cancer, cause cure and cover-up" available/orderable all bookshops.

Summary

This chapter is intended to alert patients to unusual causes of Candida. Just setting off thoughts and then being able to refer to an appropriate section may help understand why Candida can come seemingly from out of the blue.

However, this chapter is not intended to be a finite reference, since that would take a book by itself; your doctor or pharmacist might be able to provide further information on specific medications if requested, but new medications are constantly being researched, tested, licensed and prescribed. Keeping abreast of pharmaceutical knowledge and new drugs is nearly impossible.

The basic ingredients of medications are usually to be found in plants, animals, moulds, bacteria or synthetic chemicals. These, we know, have enormous influences on our body systems. When compounded, synthesised, purified and administered, they must conform to rigid pharmaceutical regulations and be proven efficient for the disease they aim to help.

Account is taken of side-effects by the manufacturer but occasional unforeseen effects do occur. Unfortunately, many do include Candidal upsurge as side effects, and whilst this may be reported when applying for a license to manufacture, it is usually underestimated, despite the fact that Candida, as we well know, can be an extremely distressing illness. Yes, it can be a minor, localised nuisance, but increasingly lasting episodes are taking time and money to disperse. Candida as a drug side-effect should be taken far more seriously by all concerned in pharmaceutical industries and by prescribing professionals. But then, perhaps they have an anti-fungal drug for sale!

6 The immune system

The immune system and immunity are misunderstood by patients and by many doctors. Yet their importance in protecting our health from industrial and commercial assault is paramount.

This book, so far, has mentioned the immune system many times in relation to other bodily systems, such as digestion, but has made no effort to describe it. Where is it? What is it? What does it do? These and other questions need to be answered in order to help us understand more.

Perhaps an analogy would be helpful. The immune system is like the moat and drawbridge of an ancient castle. There are defence towers at vantage points in the walls and battlements for firing arrows or pouring boiling oil onto attackers, and there is also a central armoury as a last bastion of defence against attack. But, of course, an atomic bomb would immediately reduce all of it to dust.

We have all these defence mechanisms. The genetics of human life are far too complex to allow death from the first bacterial, fungal or other illness to come along. Too much effort has gone into human construction to allow a quick kill. No, the human body has splendid defences against marauding bands of bacteria, fungi and illnesses. To understand something of its working and the strength of its capabilities, we also have to understand that its strength depends upon the way we look after it, since, going back to our castle analogy, without food, water, bows and arrows, water in the moat, hot oil and fresh men, the walls would quickly be climbed by attackers.

We already know that one of our means of defence against Candida upsurge in the intestines is competition between bacteria and yeasts over territory. A lack of either one in the balancing act, caused by abuse or absence of nutrients, can also dictate colony strength, upsurge and territorial gain. What of other effects on Candidal upsurge by illness, tiredness, drugs and medications? How does the human body defend against these?

The modern immune system has devolved in its genetic inheritance over millions of years to resist infection. Just as people learned to use weapons to fight external attacks, so they are provided with internal microbial, chemical and anti-toxic defence weapons to repel illness.

Our skin is practically watertight and sweat encourages impure organisms to leave if they do penetrate but oils and heavier liquids like mercury, if smeared on can become absorbed into pores. Only the mouth, nose and ears are open ducts for the intake of infections or viruses, though secondary sites are the vulval area in women (both the urethra and vagina), the tip of the penis in men and the anal opening in both sexes. The anus has the ability to close very tightly and beyond it, teeming bacteria would soon repel invasion by outsiders. Anal infections are rare.

Clothing helps as a barrier against bacterial invasion. From earliest times men and women have covered genitalia both for privacy but also as protection against injury or dirt. Despite African rituals of female circumcision supposedly to prevent sexual straying and diseases it is better to cover the vulva with loose cotton material. Male circumcision was also adopted in hot countries to reduce infection and limit odour; some men object, some men do not. However, effective retraction of the folds of the foreskin is an important aid to male urethral health and that of his sexual partner. Male circumcision may be a medical necessity for some clinical ailments but female circumcision is not so indicated.

The commonest routes of organism invasion are the mouth and nose. Sneezing is the response of ever-sifting villi hairs lining the epithelium of the airways. An intruder is captured by villi, sunk into the moist mucus and then sneezed out or coughed up. In the mouth, antibodies are constantly on the lookout for invading bacteria, as are those in the nose and throat, and they eject or disable vast numbers of bacteria, fungi, spores, cells and viruses without any trouble. Large amounts of incoming bacteria and fungi present antibodies with a problem. If, for example, you ran through a wood full of falling leaves and rotting branches, you would inhale the mould spores in massive quantities, which might cause tight breathing or even an asthma attack if you were prone to such attacks. When these sorts of situations occur and antibodies developed in past responses can't cope or cannot be reproduced in time, other responses happen. The bloodstream will transport immune system defences to the site to fight further infiltration of the invading allergen or infection.

For toxinous bacterial repulsion, phagocytes - or white blood cells, as they are also called - quickly overwhelm and usually destroy the invader; in response to mould spores, histamine, which is useful in small amounts for easing local inflammation, goes into overdrive. Unfortunately, it swings out of control in the heavy spore inhalation and goes from being effective to becoming a nuisance itself by helping to clog up airways and cause breathing difficulties. All allergy sufferers will be familiar with this. Pharmaceutical discoveries recommend anti-histamine medications to calm it down and ease the breathing by dilating bronchial tubes.

If some kind of virus, which is a complete stranger to body defences, invades, then a new, specifically relevant antibody which can mimic the cells of the invader has to be made. This can take anything from several hours to a couple of days, by which time, meeting scant resistance, the invading virus multiplies victoriously. Eventually, its relevant antibody gains ground, but maybe not before several miserable days or weeks for the host have passed. At least the genetic continuation of the host body has been assured (in other words, we won't die!). It is a kind of self-immunisation.

Nevertheless, some very intrepid bacteria manage to get past the white cells. They are classified in two groups: as exotoxins, with an ability to destroy white cells by secreting a killer protein all over the white cells, and as another group called aggressins, which help toxins to dissolve or liquify ailing body tissue. All the following bacteria belong to one of these two toxinous, damaging groups, but will respond to antibiotics when our own natural body antibiotic, called lysozyme, has been overworked.

streptococcus groups A-Q
scarlet fever due to a strep. infection
staphylococcus (also MRSA- Multiple Resistant Staph Aureus)
pneumococcus
shigella and cholera
salmonella
tetanus
diphtheria
meningococcus
syphilis
gonococcus
borrelia
mycobacterium tuberculosis and leprosy

The constant, daily, unseen invasion by bacteria and fungi is always efficiently controlled and rejected by white cells. Their activity upon an invading bacteria is called phagocytosis, but we all know or recognise when our 'central armoury' has been bombed - that is when we need antibiotic help.

Natural resistance

This ability of the protective, defending white cells and other friendly host bacteria is called 'natural resistance'. It can rise dramatically when the host body is genetically strong, eats sensibly, stays fresh, is not under stress and tired. A genetic weakness in defences , can be a lifelong problem. We all know these sorts of people. They catch anything that's going around, feel frequently tired, lack energy and are more often away from work. Of course, this may also be because they have a poor diet or 'burn the candle at both ends', but we still know people who do all the right things, yet are always 'below par'. They probably lack a strong natural resistance. Such people can only do their best to sleep properly, work at an acceptable rate, eat a well-balanced diet and stabilise this tender immune system with regular mineral and vitamin supplements. Their immune system may also be dealing with the constant 24 hour vapour from mercury teeth fillings which is toxinous. Other dental metals can also reduce immune energy and function. Beryllium, cobalt, nickel are all toxins and capable of causing mysterious bad health.

Adaptive immune response

If you have an exact repetition of an infection or virus, the immune system will recognise it, since it has invaded before. The antibody which was created to deal with the first attack will be 'called up' and will instantly begin to fight off the first few invasive cells, so that colonies are killed and further bloodstream infiltration is immediately prevented. Ever had mumps or chicken pox? Well, they never or rarely return, do they? This is also known as 'acquired resistance'. One of the earliest, medically observed episodes was of cowpox. Dr Edward Jenner, a Gloucestershire doctor in 1794, wondered why milkmaids who constantly milked cows with infected scabrous udders never seemed to get smallpox when it occasionally rampaged through local communities. Having heard of Middle Eastern stories, brought home by Lady Mary Wortley Montagu, who was a great traveller, about tribes who scraped old infection from one person into the skin of an uninfected person to protect them from the worst excess of the illness, Dr Jenner decided to conduct an experiment. He took some of the liquid weeping off the cows' udders and scratched it onto village children, none of whom contracted smallpox as a result. This was the first medical vaccination in the Western world.

Dr Jenner used live, fresh, single virus material uncontaminated by preservatives or additives. And he did not inject deep into muscle tissue nor assault small babies with it.

There are now several excellent books on what vaccination as we know it today has become. 'Vaccination' by Dr Viera Scheibner is one such and a revelation for parents and doctors who are worried by autism, behavioural problems, asthma and many childhood illnesses. The immune system of six week old babies is undeveloped and cannot withstand the assault from an injection of modern vaccine material. The baby may have immediate breathing problems often at night and many Cot deaths have been recorded on days 1-9, then 45 and 90 following vaccination. Older people pressurized into having influenza vaccine frequently report feeling ill for weeks and many never recover their former healthy sparkle. These groups have absent or ageing immune system defences and deeply injecting muscle with modern contaminated vaccine material is unhelpful to say the least, killingly harmful at the worst.

I am a convert to more natural means and in favour of keeping babies away from people and busy places where bacteria are overwhelming.

Years ago new babies were only held by their nursing mother and kept in quiet, safe surroundings. They were not taken down to the superstore and bombarded with adult germs. Nature and her immune defence are not keeping up with modern life, it is we who should defer and be more sensible. Polio vaccine caused an epidemic of disfigured limbs in the 1950's where the injection needle was inserted. It was later prescribed to be taken on a sugar lump and the disfigurement and disability stopped; I'm all for that. I want Thimerosal, the mercury preservative used to promote longer shelf life for vaccines, replaced with something less toxic and I'd like to see a complete overhaul of ingredients, additives, times and administration techniques. Our immune systems are being assaulted by modern day vaccine technology and we are suffering as a result.

Transplants, grafting and rejection

These pioneering efforts to replace damaged organs in one body with replacement organs from another still face obstinate problems of rejection. The rejection is a microbial one, an immune system failing to recognise and then fighting off a group of cells from a foreign source. Many drugs try to fight or fool the host's immune response, but failure rate is still high. Our immune systems are strongly individual and very loyal, even to the point of rejecting things that are intended to help us.

AUTO-IMMUNITY

Sometimes, because messages may be faulty or incomplete, the immune system turns upon itself rather than the incoming invasion of micro-organisms. Or perhaps it simply isn't stimulated and sits back whilst the invaders take over the host body. Worse still, the immune system can also think that normal host body organisms are actually the invaders and turn on them.

HYPERSENSITIVITY

We touched on this earlier in this chapter when we mentioned histamine. If histamine or some other chemical response is activated by an allergen like mould spores in a wood, then we hope it will work correctly. Often, unfortunately, it doesn't and flows copiously, causing reactions to itself rather than the allergenic substance. This can, if constantly repeated, damage the epithelial lining of the areas most affected - the intestine if it's a food allergy, the Eustachian tube if it's an ear problem, the nasal cavities if it's an allergic rhinitis or the trachea (wind pipe) and lungs if it's an asthmatic reaction. As the years go by, these areas become 'boggy' or sponge-like. The problem worsens, and steroid drugs prescribed to make life bearable may cause additional side-effects like Candida.

IMMUNITY TO CANDIDA AND OTHER YEASTS

The immune system has a regulatory control process for fungi as well as bacteria, viruses and parasites. As with the latter, fungi also extend their involvement in a host body by genetic inheritance. Sensitivity is also influenced strongly by additional health problems, tiredness, drugs and medication, dietary quality, diabetes, hormonal levels, anaemia, old age or immuno-depression. In other words, lowered resistance and damage. Apart from Candida Albicans, other fungi should be mentioned here:

- **Pneumocystis Carinii** is present as a severe complication of HIV Aids
- **Histoplasma, Coccidioides** and **Blastomyces** can all cause fungal infections of the lungs;
- **Cryptococcus** is another yeast often upsurging in severely ill patients.

The latter can take hold in the meninges (membrane surrounding the spinal cord and brain) and in the brain and can be extremely serious. Aspergillus and Actinomycetes are all able to cause lung difficulties and malaise. Some are found in horses' stables and hay.

Candida Albicans

We know that this is present already in our bodies. It lives harmlessly in the intestines, but can also be found inhabiting the vagina, mouth, throat, ears, nasal cavities - in fact, any moist membranous area. Patients already ill and usually in hospital will have blood tests taken for Candida. Deficiencies or defects in **T cells** and polymorphs (PMN) are notable, and the next section discusses the cell systems responsible for immunity. I personally see no reason why such blood tests, or reviseable cheaper versions, cannot also be made available to those who, this century, have been immune-damaged by diet or drugs.

In 1943, a study on genetic responsibility as a possible reason for Candida lesions in three related children showed an endocrine malfunction identical in all three of them. Further studies showed a lymphocyte function failure and even that Candida itself suppresses the immune system, leading to a cycle of events that further weakens the host. A lymphocyte is a cell in the bloodstream which adapts to incoming intruders, even if it is not the specific antibody. It travels in and out of the lymph glands, which are tiny, bean-shaped nodules in various parts of the body. They usually swell up in fevers or malaise, indicating poor health. Lymphocytes help fight infections and are carried in lymph, a milky liquid carried in lymphatic vessels, much like blood vessels (veins and arteries) transport blood.

T AND B LYMPHOCYTES

There are several types of lymphocytes, including T, B and PMN. T lymphocytes originate in the Thymus glands at the base of the neck. Their function is to recognise intruders and adapt, if necessary, to kill viruses, control fungi and clear dead cells from host tissues. B lymphocytes secrete antibodies which again help to recognise and fight invaders. They, too, are very adaptive in their ability to do this. If antigens (stimulators) of antibody production are deficient in some way, then T and **B cells** may be less able to adapt. T and B cells closely interact with each other, and there may be several reasons for a diminished function or response.

PMN (polymorphonuclear) is another important lymphocyte. It contains granules which are very powerful killers of bacteria by enzyme activity. Some of these enzymes may be gene damaged and contribute to fungal infections.

In 1968, another important paper by Buckley and colleagues showed defective responses to Candida Albicans by lymphocyte cells. Clearly the intricate liaisons, or interaction, between these lymphocytes and fungal control is important. If the genetic inheritance (gene malfunction causing a predisposition to above-average or regular upsurges of Candida) dictates events and leads to lymphocyte malfunction (as observed in studies of family Candida), then a most important area of cause is determined, which requires more study.

OTHER CULPRITS

How often have I heard women say that they take all possible precautions via self-help, yet one apple/cake/glass of wine will bring them down. If there is no diabetes, no drug damage, no other illness, no poor diet, etc., then we must look to something else, somewhere else. There are other factors.

Of the specific cells which give rise to natural immunity rather than the adaptive qualities of the lymphocytes, these are some worth a mention for our purposes.

- Lysozyme and interferon are the 'natural' antibiotics of the immune system. Their antibacterial qualities fight bacterial invasions by attacking bacterial cell walls. Once this happens, the contents leak out of the membrane and the intruder cell dies.
- MAC (macrophage) cells then dispose of the dying, damaged or dead cells.
- Phagocytosis is the action of the MAC and PMN cells. Almost all of the dead rubbish is removed by this action.

If there is too much *natural* antibiotic activity and not enough debris clearance, then fungi are attracted. Too much antibacterial activity may decrease the vital balancing act between bacteria and yeasts, leaving the ideal conditions for optimum yeast surge; if debris from dead cells is not collected and ejected, yeasts may well seize upon this additional, rotting nutrition.

Studies of fungal activity accounted for much of the activity of the large pharmaceutical companies in the 1990s. Since antibiotic therapy has reached a plateau of success, attention is turning to treatments for Candida and other fungi. In the process of formulating ideas for new drugs to treat the variety of upsurge points, like skin, gut, vagina, nasal cavities, scientists will need to spend a great deal of time in looking at spores in detail. Since bacteria in the body tend to be controlled by other bacteria, then it is possible that fungal upsurge of one kind could be controlled by a different competing kind of fungus.

At some stage someone may well uncover the intricacies of internal fungus-to-fungus control mechanisms. About one and a half million species of fungi exist worldwide. Perhaps a competent drug from one of them will not only be developed as a medication, but also prove to be present already in small amounts within the immune system. There are some accepted anti-fungal drugs which work well enough, though neither scientists, doctors nor patients are entirely happy with them. We will discuss anti-fungal drugs later on.

Other immune responses

It is not only bacteria and fungi that are controlled by an active, healthy immune system. We should mention some other diseases which respond either permanently or in part to immune control.

VIRUSES

Rubella (Measles)

Herpes viruses
Includes simplex, varicella, cytomegalovirus, EBV strains.

- The cold sore strain can frequently recur during stress and can be transmitted. It is controllable by a daily tablet of Lysine (available at any chemist) at the onset of an upsurge.
- Varicella (chicken pox). This never recurs as chicken pox, though it may recur in the form of shingles (zoster).
- EBV is an infectious virus which may generate into Burkitt's Lymphoma, a malignant lymph cancer.
- CMV is an infection which commonly appears in patients whose immune system is suppressed, usually by drugs or severe illness.

Rhinoviruses and Adenoviruses
Cause colds and sore throats, and are always adapting; immunity to them is almost unattainable.

Enteroviruses
These viruses, which include polio, wreak havoc before the immune system has time to find antibodies.

Hepatitis
Affects the liver; is either of A strain, which is infectious, B strain, which is introduced into the bloodstream from infected needles and contaminated blood transfusions or the newly discovered C strain.

Retroviruses
Usually deadly. They include leukaemia virus types and HIV.

Myxoviruses
Include influenza of all sorts, measles and mumps.

Foreign viruses

These include Lassa Fever, Kurn, Typhus, Yellow Fever and Rabies and may need vaccination to give better protection. Check the preservative first, refuse Thimerosal.

PARASITES

There are four groups of parasitic illnesses determined by the means of entry into the host body.

Water and food

These can carry Entamoeba, Toxoplasma, Giardia, Balantidium, Cryptosporidium and Isospora, which all cause malaise, diarrhoea, dysentery and nausea. They do better when the host body is already immuno depleted, but can be contracted in areas of contamination. Giardia, for instance, is currently common in German, Russian, Eastern Baltic States and other European water supplies. Outbreaks occur in Britain from time to time. Whilst prescribed antibiotics do not always effect relief, Paramycrocidin, Citricidin or grapefruit extract supplements do. Ask your pharmacist to look up suppliers; don't touch alcohol, red meat, coffee, tea or ice-cream for as long as it takes - maybe months if the parasite has gained a real hold. Constantly check out emerging products from any background.

Insect bites

These can cause malaria of several types from mosquitoes; Trypanosoma gambiense and rhodesiense (sleeping sickness) from tsetse flies in African countries; Leishmania carried by sandflies; Lyme Disease; Babesia carried by cattle ticks; Trypanosoma cruzi or Chagas' disease from bugs found on cattle drinking at infected water holes in Central or South America. There are lots more where these come from!

Opportunist invasion

Invasion by parasites, such as Pneumocystis and Toxoplasma, can also add significantly to illnesses already suffered.

Antigenic variation

Variation of some parasite effects can decrease severity of returning symptoms, as in malaria or the trypanosome groups.

WORMS

These common parasites have plagued humans and animals since time began. They and their eggs abound in soil and water, and they can become uncontrollable, especially in areas of low hygiene and high humidity. They can spread from small children, animals and those working on the land. Scrubbing finger nails, drinking purified water, changing towels and nightwear each day are essential. Medication has to be taken by everyone in the home and should be taken daily for as long as necessary. This combats the lengthy and rampant life cycle of the worm.

There are all sorts of round worms, tapeworms and flukes. Stool samples will disclose which sort is present and medication must begin immediately. We have no natural immunity to worms, nor do we appear able to acquire any. Possibly our immune system exercises a small degree of control, but certainly not in sufficient force to defeat the intruders. Humans and animals have always been plagued by worms.

TUMOURS

Studies of non-malignant and malignant cancers abound. Thousands of scientists vie with each other and their competitive groups to make significant advances in this field of medicine. Immune response to cancer cells is a vital area of work, but too complicated to go into here. However, it is known that macrophages and killer cells within the natural immune response can prevent some kinds of tumours growing in laboratory conditions. In animal studies, they have even been able to kill cancerous cells. So work on enhancing cells and functions within our own immunity to kill life-threatening cancer invasions is an exciting advance. Even surgical procedures are declining due to advances in chemo- and radiotherapy advances. Antibodies and T-cell responses are some other areas being focused on by scientists worldwide. It's an exciting race, but the differing cancers require diverse treatments and immune responses, so overnight breakthroughs are unlikely.

Excellent books on cancer by Dr Hulda Clark and Ron Gdanski are ground-breaking in diagnosing and treating cancers without surgery. Since cancers occur mostly in membrane walls of storage vessels and ducts such as lungs, colon, breast, prostate, lymph system, they suggest that nutritional deficiencies, bacterial infections, chemical toxins, viral growths, physical injury and parasites may be responsible. They say that cancer is the 'continuous multiplication, mutation and rejection of membrane cells that fail to repair an injury'. Their ground-breaking research and books deal with all sorts of cancers and give details of immune system support through lifestyle changes.

ALLERGIES

Whether or not doctors and scientists have taken allergies seriously in the past, they do now. Environmentally, our air is now full of allergens from industry and lifestyle. Breathing difficulties, digestive disorders are common reactions to certain foods/ drinks/inhalants/fumes/seasons/climate/substances. It may also seem clear to many sufferers that allergies tend to run in families but such a perceived inheritance may be due to other unknown factors.

Even though science has now identified a gene in DNA that is responsible for some genetic asthma and rhinitis (runny nose), these conditions are also known to be caused by mercury vapour from teeth fillings and fillings are commonplace! More discoveries are sure to follow. Horizons of allergenic response may need to be broadened. Why should there only be a lung, sinus or skin rash reaction to any substance? We know that food allergies are common - for instance, peanuts, cereal products and dairy products - which are readily accepted by every doctor. But if you grant that even these exist, then, by extension, it is also possible for a wider variety to be acknowledged.

In studies of Candida as an allergen, mice have been seen to produce histamine as a response to Candida introduction, and follow-up studies found the same in guinea pigs, monkeys and tested humans. As far back as 1920, papers have been published on skin inflammation response to Candidal skin eruptions. Doctors specialising in Candida trials found that patients responded completely when treated for psoriasis, urticaria and dermatitis with anti-fungal medications. This, they felt, was a vindication of the diagnosis that, for many such patients, Candida Albicans was responsible. They also found evidence of Saccharomyces Cerevisiae, the brewer/ baker/distillery yeast in patients with urticaria (also known as hives; an itchy, raised, inflamed patch of skin which often occurs in clusters).

For Candida sufferers and their doctors, immunity to, or immune-sensitivity to Candida is very much an up-and-coming research area. Immunologists working in the field may be interested in patients with an apparent lifelong disposition to Candidosis.

7 Sufferers and symptoms

Doubtless many people will find it strange that the explanation of the symptoms of Candida and a review of those who suffer them are placed so far into the book. However, anyone leafing through this book in the bookshop will either be a sufferer looking for help or a browser. The latter will put it back quickly, but the former will be far more likely to know the symptoms already. Nevertheless, I think it is important that we should not only review many of the more commonly known symptoms now, but also be made aware of the great variety of them. Medications and treatments will be discussed in later chapters.

Symptoms of vaginal thrush/yeast infection

There are two distinct types of vaginal thrush.

The commonest is known by heat; redness; vulval swelling; heavy, stringy, creamy vaginal discharge; irritation, ranging from mild discomfort through to near-phobic scratching, especially at night; odour; unbearably painful response to any sexual intercourse; variable levels of anal irritation (Pruritis Ani); low pelvic aching; spreading inflammatory redness along the perineum, maybe even down the thighs; great irritation of pubic hair follicles; possibly painful urination, cystitis; any attempts to scratch or rub may produce sexual orgasm.

The second type, not always understood as vaginal thrush, is when there is Candida involvement elsewhere at the same time. The situation in the vagina is an outward sign of the situation in the intestines and bowels. There is severe swelling; a purple-reddening of the vulva, whose two entrances (urethra and vagina) appear almost closed up; vaginal and vulval dryness may lead to skin cracks which are agonising; micturition (passing urine) may be painful and hesitant; walking may be painful and exercise impossible; sexual intercourse will be impossible; general lethargy adds to the misery and then there is that attendant smell! Lichenised patches may occur in the pubic hair follicles. These will be very sensitive and itchy. Each patch will dry out and slough off the dead skin flecks. Alternatively, scratching may cause clear or bloody exudation. Again, orgasm can result from rubbing or scratching.

SUFFERERS OF VAGINAL THRUSH

Although it is mainly women who suffer from vaginal thrush, babies and little girls can, too. In dealing with vaginal thrush, we see an immediately similar situation going on an inch or so away at the anus. Both places have a sympathetic balance of Candida with appropriate bacteria. If swabs of a normal vagina are taken, they show very low numbers of quite a wide variety of micro-organisms, but this flora depends heavily upon the usual requirements of warmth, nutrients and correctly balanced **pH**. Warmth is taken for granted, except when it swings to a higher heat from exercise or cooler, as perhaps when sitting in the snow. It is the amount of nutrients and the acid/alkaline balance which matter. We shall discuss our own influence in controlling these later when we deal with self-help.

Pruritis ani (itchy anus) obviously has a greater colonisation of anal surfaces. Intestinal bacteria exit from here in faeces, having probably passed some time in the rectal cavity (bowels), where multiplication continues. Haemorrhoidal veins will swell and itch and possibly even bleed. The numbers of Candida spores exiting the anus and then remaining on the perineum add to those already in the vagina which were probably originally deposited from initial faecal residue transfer. Any upsurge in faecal numbers or any lapse in efficient control of them can result in vaginal upsurge.

By far the commonest causes of Candidal vaginal upsurge are those which have been self-induced. They include heavy sugar intake (which acts as a nutrient for the Candida); one or more courses of antibiotics taken for any infection in the body; diabetes and high sugar levels in both bloodstream and urine; raised body temperatures from excessive exercising; alcohol; swimming in chlorinated or antiseptic pools; wearing tight or non-porous clothing; failing to take action before and after menstruation to counteract alkalinity; sexual transmittance (including oral sex); poor hygiene.

Having listed these main causes, it should be said that many other personal factors can add to trouble, but most will fall into one of the above-mentioned areas of self-caused upsurges. It is an uncomfortable fact that few women never get vaginal thrush; that lots of women have several attacks over a lifetime; and that vaginal thrush is the commonest women's vaginal problem. In those unfortunates who suffer early in life, upsurges are likely to recur time and again, if prevention has been ignored.

Whilst the condition is prevalent in women between the ages of eighteen and forty-five, it can be a plague to older women, who may then go on to experience reduced insulin and pancreatic function leading to disordered sugar synthesis as part of ageing. Old age also brings stiffening joints which can make maintenance of good perineal hygiene difficult. Wrists and hips find increasing difficulty with bending, turning and cleaning the perineum.

OTHER OBSERVATIONS

Candida has an ability to stick onto the walls of the vagina, but this can vary according to oestrogenic influences and to any lasting effects from frequent past upsurges. This will happen when hyphae (the threadlike filaments on the fungus) have not only adhered to but penetrated cell walls. Such a situation tends to occur when women are failing to observe the stringent self-help rules and are allowing development of a welcoming environment for Candida, rather than removing all its preferences.

There is also evidence now of deficient T lymphocyte responses in vaginal Candidosis. Immune responses may not be fully activated to repel attempts by Candida to adhere and colonise. There may be a blockage in lymphocytes' response to invasion by macrophage secretions of prostaglandin. There may also be antibody malfunction suppressing T lymphocyte activity.

Some research into vaginal Candida as an allergen in hypersensitive women has shown elevations of IgE, the antibody which causes breakdown of the mast cells (the cells that release histamine). It is frequently seen in allergy sufferers.

Whilst doctors and researchers have associated increased glycogen in the vagina with hormonal changes, as in menstrual cycles and pregnancy, which affect vaginal pH, some current thinking claims a lack of sufficient scientific proof to back this. Most women with premenstrual cyclical thrush recurring time and again may well feel that they have proof enough! Lactic acid pessaries or a rinse-out with a mild solution of cider vinegar and water ease and control the alkaline fungal upsurge without recourse to doctors and drugs.

Symptoms of penile Candida

The first description of thrush of the penis was in 1920, and medical statistics of the incidence of penile symptoms have been poorly kept. When there is a problem, symptoms include soreness, redness, some irritation, sore urination, perhaps a drop or two of unusually whitish discharge, white spots or lesions under the foreskin. Alcoholics or diabetics can have permanent trouble and, more noticeably, a lot of burping and passing of wind. Penile thrush can be transmitted during intercourse and may worsen from the heat generated by thrusting.

SUFFERERS OF THRUSH OF THE PENIS

Of course, dietary factors, immunity, strength, allergenic response, clothing, illness, diabetes and sugary drinks all affect men, too, but in general, thrush troubles men far less than women, even when they have it. Those seeming to be more at risk are diabetics, heavy drinkers, smokers, men whose sexual partner is a regular thrush sufferer, HIV Aids victims and cancer patients, but all other reasons, such as antibiotics, can equally apply. Penile thrush is sexually transmittable.

Candida of the urethra, bladder and kidneys

URETHRA

This is barely, if at all, recognised by the average general practitioner. Faeces carry intestinal bacteria and yeasts on the railroad route from anus to vulva. Toilet paper is microscopically insufficient to remove them, only effective washing will.

In women, simple walking spreads the organisms along. The more there are, the faster they will move inwards. Before a menstrual period alkalinity in the vagina accepts yeasts readily and the adjacent urethral opening may also be alkaline. Even the urethral epithelium will, with its normally mild and well-washed habitat, be unable to put up a fight against energetic forays by yeasts. On the other hand, there may only be a reactive twingeing in the urethra, not a real infestation. Both male and female urethras, in spite of the differences in length, can receive additional spores to those normally in-dwelling, not just from sexual transference, but also from contaminated underwear.

In general, men are less aware of the need to use an acceptable amount of toilet paper. Should heavy faecal residues with high levels of yeasts and bacteria chance to come into contact with the tip of the penis, transference to underwear may occur.

Whilst women have a separate urethra lying alongside the vagina, men have one tube doing two jobs. Both urine and semen flow down the urethral tube which, in men, is more elastic to enable an erection to occur. Some studies into prostatitis caused by Candida show that not only might male fertility be reduced because sperm cannot move around easily, but that in some cases prostate abscesses may have Candida as a cause. These studies also show that Candida is quite capable of moving up the length of the male urethra to colonise in the prostate gland. New interest and studies show Mycoplasma genitalium present in prostate infection.

BLADDER

As with all latest ideas, investigations and research studies, the more people learn, the more they realise they don't know. There appears to be very little research into bladder Candida in contrast to the stronger probability that much cystitis, urethritis/non-specific urethritis may indeed be due to Candida or Mycobacteria, if only tests were undertaken or requested to prove it. From urine samples of people with cystitis who fail to show either a bacterial or non-bacterial cause for continuous pain, heat and stinging micturition, a higher than average count of yeasts on culture plates can be found. Many immuno-compromised patients have serious infestations in their urine. Also teeming with yeasts are urine samples from patients who have been catheterised or have urinary catheters in place.

Yeasts can be detected in a urine sample as bacteria, provided the microbiologist has been requested to find them. Culture plates provide nutrients, whilst hot shelves mimic the 37C body temperature which Candida species of all sorts enjoy. However, a biopsy of the site may be more reliable. Whilst family doctors readily understand the use of swabs for vaginal and penile samples and know that swabs for Candida can be taken, many seem to have forgotten the use of urine samples and biopsies for proving yeasts in the bladder.

Mycoplasma and Ureaplasma are increasingly seen with correct analysis to be responsible for so-called Interstitial Cystitis where there is 24/7/12 bladder pain. The very strong and lengthy course of antibiotics needed to see off this intransigent bacterial form will cause Candida so take an anti-fungal afterwards.

(See: The Patient's Encyclopaedia of Cystitis, Sexual Cystitis, Interstitial Cystitis. www.angela.kilmartin.dial.pipex.com   or any book shop)

KIDNEYS

Candida can also be detected in the bloodstream (one test is called the Isolator). Other ways of finding Candida in the blood are by radiometry or using substances such as charcoal and certain resins. So precise are the conditions required for accurate sample taking that you may be requested to attend the microbiology department itself so that a microbiologist can draw the blood and set up the blood culture bottles. These bloodstream tests are not widely used, partly for the precision in preparation, but also because of the costs. Results may take anything up to two weeks, and even then may be completely false due to a variety of current test inadeqacies.

Once within the bloodstream, yeasts are nurtured in the alkaline environment, and deposition may commence in the kidneys. From an infested bladder, there is also the probability that Candida will progress up each ureter to the kidneys to utilise a secondary route of transference. There is considerable scientific data on Candidosis of the kidneys (although little actual documentation), but diagnosis through tests is only recommended on seriously immuno-suppressed patients. If they are known to be immuno-suppressed, then it will be assumed that Candidosis is present anyway in the patient.   More women than men or children contract Candidosis of the kidneys, and, of these, it is most common in women over fifty who have a history of urinary troubles like cystitis or nephritis, and diabetes. Candida seems to settle and obstruct kidney or ureter function by forming balls of fungus, so retention of urine may be an additional help in diagnosis, though urinary retention in the bladder can be caused by different factors.

Babies and children are equally prone to Candidosis of the kidney and urinary tract. For some, breast-feeding may be the route of transmission or nappies may harbour yeasts and infest the vulva or penis; a seriously sick or pre-term baby is just as likely to contract Candidosis as someone older, since its immune system is under stress.

Although renal Candidosis is sparsely documented, this does not mean that there are few sufferers. Given money, accurate tests and an alert doctor, it is highly likely that larger numbers of patients would emerge in the general practice community. Once Candida is in situ elsewhere in vital organs of a sick body, it can also be found in the kidneys because blood carries it there.

Treatment can vary according to the site, but systemic drugs, such as Sporanox, fluconazole or flucytosine are best, though there are others. Painful installations of anti-fungal liquids into the bladder may be suggested and should be refused. Sporanox should not be prescribed for pregnant women.

I must say that my research for this book has left me staggered at the amount of data proving Candida as an extremely well-documented, whole-body condition. It doesn't only affect the vagina in women or the mouth in babies - or between toes, where most primary healthcare professionals accept it, so why is systemic Candida so unaccepted?

The more I uncover, the more I wonder whether general practice is kept in the dark on purpose by the researchers and training hospitals, yet I can think of no good reason why this could be. There is no doubt that diagnostic blindness affects many frontline professionals who fail to acknowledge that Candidal involvement is every bit as serious as bacterial infections.

Candida of the skin

Sufferers include everyone as possible candidates. Although Candida Parapsilosis and Candida Guilliermondii can be found on skin, it is still Candida Albicans which heads the list. Favoured sites are feet because they are dark, sweaty and warm from wearing shoes like trainers; warm, sweaty crotches encased in tights, leotards, sportswear and non-breathing materials; the folds of finger skin from regular immersion in water remaining warm and moistened. Tight bracelets, watch straps, non-porous clothing, gloves or footwear, whether for sports or the workplace, create patches and areas of warmth and moisture which attract skin-based Candida spores. Sweat anywhere, with all its moist nutrients, provides a habitat which promotes Candidal growth. Larger female breasts can harbour Candida underneath and should be washed, dried and powdered regularly.

The area between our legs is dark, warm, moist and covered up by clothing. Candida may also find a home in the groin where folds of skin from the lower abdomen, especially in obese people, touch the inner thighs. Air is again excluded, and heat with sweat encourages fungal growth. This is more likely to occur in climates which are already warm and moist, though the wearing of incorrect clothing in a cold climate, where fierce room heating is present, can also create sweat.

Babies are susceptible to nappy rash, with Candida as an isolated organism. This can be caused by the modern use of plastic linings/grips/polyester-type absorbents and the external plastic material. All of the nappy excludes air. As a result, a thriving market in creams, lotions, medicated wipes and powders has grown to reduce the formation and settlement of fungal spores. Whenever the weather or climate is favourable, either indoors or out, exposure to air is very helpful for such troubled babies.

Many other skin rashes, like eczema, psoriasis, urticaria, acne, some spots with pus heads and scalp irritations, may, if cultured, show Candida as a dominating organism. Scrapings from the affected area are easily obtained and cultured in a laboratory if requested.

Candidal infestation of the finger nails is more frequently seen than in toe nails. Again, the predominant social factors are jobs where hands are kept wet for long periods. Nail infestations can also be a side-effect in people with peripheral vascular disease; Cushings Syndrome; people who use steroid creams under elastoplast dressings and people who wash frequently with harsh liquids or antiseptics.

Fungal ear infections are increasingly seen by alert doctors in general practice and maybe found in conjunction with an ingrained infection such as Staphylococcus Aureus. Intense, weeping irritation is easily collected on a cotton swab stick and sent for culture if requested. Dry irritation cannot be collected.

There are appropriate treatments for specific sites of skin fungal infestations, yet the underlying cause always needs to be addressed. If an occupation or sport is responsible, adaptation or change may be necessary to prevent fungal outbreaks. The constant administration of anti-fungal creams is at best costly and at worst irresponsible if underlying factors can be prevented and removed instead.

SYMPTOMS OF SKIN CANDIDA

There is usually some form of irritation; this may be pus heads on spots; some kinds will even be crusted, appearing as blackened, scabrous exudations; finger nails cease to grow and become white and deadened; inflammation and redness extend around the site; most sites are moist and sticky. Scratching will simply spread it further on site as well as transferring it to other sites via the finger nails.

Candida in the eyes

An autopsy of an eye in 1943 provided the first written evidence of Candida in this site. Further post-mortems followed, showing retina damage, but not until scientific data was collected in the 1960s did Candida in the eyes become verifiable in living people. This kind of infestation is primarily blood-borne, though instances of external introduction are documented. Sometimes this external introduction has been a result of eye surgery, where contaminated instruments or bowls of fluids left exposed in unsuitable storage conditions have been proven transmitters.

SUFFERERS

Can include sufferers from intestinal Candida; patients having had abdominal surgery; drug addicts; very sick patients; immuno-compromised patients; people in intensive care or elsewhere on intravenous drips; catheterised patients; babies on intravenous drips; and varying permutations of these situations. Documentation of Candida in the eyes is now beyond doubt.

SYMPTOMS

These include blurred vision caused by lesions on the retina; some pain; examination of the affected retina shows discharge of varying colours between white, cream or yellow; reddened lesions of the iris and lens; occasional bleeding into the white of the eyes.

Proving the existence of Candida in the eye involves not only a history-take by medical personnel, but also swab and blood cultures. If other sites show past or present Candida, from stool, ear, mouth, vagina or elsewhere, it is much more likely that it is also in the eyes, either or both. Several of the Candida species may be individually responsible for lesions in eyes. Mercury attaches to the retina and may allow fungus to grow since normal immune response for keeping the eye healthy may be occupied with removing the mercury. Candida may responsively get to creep in.

Treatment for Candida is by drops and/or orally, since other areas may well be affected. There are several topical preparations which help, including flucytosine and any of the amphotericins. Treatment for removal of mercury is by sulfur drops to which mercury binds and is ejected.

Candida in deep organ tissue

By deep organ tissue, I mean the outer and inner construction of all the main organs of the body. These are brain, lungs, heart, liver and kidneys. Smaller organs are just as much at risk and some have already been discussed. Professor Odds in his book states that 'systemic Candida infections continue to constitute a significant medical problem'. This may well mean a rising incidence because of several factors:

- In days gone by, the life of the patient wouldn't have been prolonged by drugs from the initial outbreak of illness. This illness would have killed quite early on, and a Candida takeover would have insufficient time to develop as a serious systemic response.
- Seriously sick patients remaining alive can now be tested for Candida.
- Increasing data storage and testing facilities mean that more cases can be discovered.
- HIV Aids is an obvious, well-observed example, but most terminally ill patients of either sex are on antibiotics, steroids, drips and multiple drugs anyway, all of which have their side-effects.
- From books, leaflets and articles, patients are themselves far more aware of Candida as an illness and are ready and willing to request the tests or at least have a discussion about it.

For Candida of any species to be proven in deep organ tissue, the history-take, past cultures, knowledge of depletive health conditions and the blood cultures are, at present, the only means of assessing whether systemic Candida is the cause of the symptoms. Only when a cheap and accurate blood test or some other kind of whole-body test is available will doctors be able to diagnose confidently and patients be relieved of frustration and suffering. There is a race on to provide such a test, but since Candida is a relative newcomer to the scientific scene, following on from bacterial infections, it may take some considerable time yet to catch up.

Candida of the mouth and throat

Sufferers are drawn from any age group or either sex. As with Pruritis Ani at the other end of the body, thrush at the top end is entirely visible. It has therefore been noted and documented for several thousand years. The additional term, apthae, was the word chosen by Hippocrates for the condition in babies' mouths, and in a 1784 book, Dr Underwood refers to this ancient term as well as the better known thrush. He described it well.

'There are white specks inside the mouth from lips to gullet, and it is said to extend the whole length of the intestines.'

He distinguishes between light, localised cases and those which 'excoriate parts of the anus'. He also observed that indigestion seemed to be a feature, possibly from 'bad milk' or 'unwholesome food'.

Dr Underwood had seen recommendations for opening the baby's bowels, cleaning the mouth out well and also giving an emetic to cause vomiting. He, himself, felt this was all a bit much for 'a tender infant', so his personal treatment plan was for mixtures called 'testacious powders' derived from magnesia or contrayerva, followed up by rhubarb to 'carry down the scales as they fall off'. The poor baby was then purged with Heister, followed by more testacious powders, camomile tea or tinctura amara. More knowingly, he goes on to pay attention to the diet of the wet nurse (a woman who, by going from one family to another, kept her own supply of breast milk flowing and earned a reasonable living by feeding other women's babies). He particularly wanted a decrease in her 'usual amount of porter or ale'! Breast milk and uncovered teats on bottles can transmit Candida directly into the baby. He added:

'A hundred different lotions and gargles have been invented for this to heal the raw wounds left by sloughed off thrush in the mouth or anus, but I have been frequently distressed at seeing a nurse rub the mouth of a little infant with a rag mop 'til she has made it bleed several times a day!'

Thrush of the mouth is also seen as white spots or plaques in all age groups, but mostly in the elderly, whose eating habits are less nutritional. Seriously sick and dying patients with systemic Candida are much troubled by swollen lips and tongue often simply looking brown and dried-out. Swallowing is an effort, since saliva production is affected too.

Older people with false teeth are often at risk from Candida colonising the gums and the roof of the mouth where the plate rests. Toothbrushes will harbour Candida and should be changed frequently. Teats, dentures and toothbrushes may be boiled in plain water.

The arrival of anti-histamine sprays for rhinitis, hay fever or asthma has brought with it a high increase in thrush of the mouth and throat. These sprays contain steroids (see chapter 5). If desensitising injections are in any way possible, they should be considered, and if moving house would remove the patient from the discovered environmental cause, then this, too, should be considered.

Hygiene is an essential help in combating thrush of the mouth, though once again the body may be immuno-depleted. Anti-fungal pastilles are available both on prescription and over the counter. Symptoms of thrush at oral sites can vary:

- ulcers and abscesses in the mouth;
- black and hairy tongue;
- brownish, dried-up tongue;
- white, raised patches inside the cheeks;
- crusted lesions at the corners of the mouth;
- inflamed and sore palate on the roof of the mouth;
- ulceration of the tongue;
- white spots around the gums;
- dry mouth and throat with difficulty in swallowing.

Thrush may be simply superficial or it may develop more deeply beyond the outer epithelium. All material involved with eating, drinking, washing or drying, cleaning teeth, dentures, etc. can harbour thrush, so be quite stringent. Choose items that can be boiled after each use.

Candida in joints or bones

Symptoms are similar to osteomyelitis and arthritis, with aching or painful joints making movement awkward. Bonded, vapourising mercury from teeth fillings can also cause such troubles. There may be inflammation and swelling with sufferers comprising two groups as specified by the route of infiltration:

- those who, through infected injections, received Candida directly into the limb;
- those who are already ill with Candidosis systemically and whose limbs become at risk.

The largest group of sufferers by far is men, and the dominant age group is between fifty and seventy years old. All sufferers, including men, women and children, from the first group probably received the fungus during surgical operations, drug infections of all sorts, including additive drugs, or tumour aspiration. Knees, jaws, shoulders, backbone, ribs and hips are the main common areas, with Candida Albicans clearly ahead of other Candida species.

For patients in the second group, there is still a male preponderance of sufferers from Candida in joints and bones, with the greatest age risk being thirty to fifty years old. Most sufferers are already low with Candidaemia - whole body infiltration - which arises out of serious illnesses, such as leukaemia and lupus of the lungs, but drug addicts and surgical cases are also notable sufferers.

Children suffering from meningitis also appear at risk from Candida in bones or joints. Other serious childhood illnesses may also be a background factor.

In nearly all cases, the Candida infiltration in bone material seems to disperse of its own accord once the patient begins to recover from the affecting background illness. Those lingering cases apparently respond well to the usual anti-fungal medications.

Candida at other sites

Simply put, this energetic fungus can penetrate everywhere. It is frequently introduced during needle injections or surgery; it is able to proliferate when the patient is low from serious illness. It may be found in the liver, any cancer sites, burns, transplants, blood transfusions, armpits, legs, blood, nerve supplies, lungs, bronchial tubes, blood vessels, heart, and all the parts of the body which have had specific attention in this chapter.

It is able to stick to moist mucosal areas throughout the body; to extend its hyphae (filaments) into tissues; to gather nutrients for its own energy requirements and to recognise when the body's immunity is lowered. It is all around us both in air we breathe and things we touch or eat.

It is still barely recognised in modern general practice except in babies' mouths, the vagina and penis, the throat and ears, hands and feet, those very sick or dying. Hippocrates and many before him knew more about Candida!

I believe that the rest of this enormous jigsaw of missing diagnoses must be addressed in our training hospitals. In between thrush in babies and genitals, or the very sick and dying, there are clearly strengths of Candidal upsurge elsewhere which need recognition. As with pre-diabetes, which is the forerunner to fully diagnosable diabetes, there may be a similar situation for Candida which needs acceptance, quicker diagnosis and faster treatment. Why wait or scorn those patients who knowledgeably feel that Candida may be their problem? Patients read their patient handbooks and self-help guides. It's time for many doctors to catch up.

8 Alternative medicine

The lack of knowledge and understanding of Candida amongst conventional Western medical practitioners has added immense frustration to long-suffering patients and it should come as no surprise that many have resorted to other forms of diagnosis and help. Of all the reasons why patients visit alternative practitioners, repetitive Candida ranks among the highest. Many patients have enormous difficulty in persuading conventional doctors of their disease, and the unavailability of cheap tests particularly for systemic candida is a great drawback. Doctors like to see confirmation of diseases, not just through symptoms but also by samples. Patients, too, want an accurate diagnosis, but when doctors are unaware that tests are appropriate at many different Candida sites, great misery and frustration is endured. Some headway is being made to find and promote easier, cheaper tests, but they may take a lot of time to become part of general practice diagnostic armoury. Until then, the patient 's own natural ability to self diagnose from a book like this is probably the best guide.

Since 1993, pharmaceutical companies manufacturing anti-fungal medications, from pastilles, pessaries and topical creams or liquids through to the strong, systemic oral treatments, have been freed, for certain products, from the list of prescriptive drugs. Anti-Candida pessaries are now available in pharmacies but are not cheap. At present - and probably in the future, too - Western countries will not want to allow oral courses of anti-fungal drugs to be de-regulated. Medical livelihoods are at stake!

I always find it mystifying that Africa, Asia, the Middle and Far East and other places are quite happy to fill pharmacy shelves with a vast array of prescribable medications which can be bought there, yet we patients who are in theory more familiar with drugs, cannot be allowed greater buying power here. My local pharmacy has shelves full of all kinds of help in tubs, bottles, packets and tubes that can help a patient to by-pass the surgery on OTC (Over the Counter) products. With assistance from the pharmacist it is possible to obtain an appropriate OTC medication for many ailments.

Arguments for further de-regulation on prescribable drugs are active between governments and pharmaceutical companies, but I believe that any further steps will be very cautious. Personally, I would like de-regulation, having been able to benefit from it for seven years in Africa and the Middle East. I can see that mistakes can be made and perhaps many would defend the status quo because of such mistakes, but it is in medical and healthcare politics where I believe the real reasons for continued regulation arise.

If Candida sufferers are denied both an attentive, knowledgable medical practitioner and immediate access to non-prescribable de-regulated drugs, then they frequently have no choice but to seek help elsewhere. Look down any health book shelf in libraries or bookshops and you will immediately become aware of the proliferation of alternative therapies. I once tried acupuncture for my allergic rhinitis, but the acupuncturist and myself conceded defeat after eight sessions. I also had six sessions of colonic irrigation to see whether this would ease the constipation which was a feature of the mercury amalgam toxicity/allergy reaction, to no lasting effect because my basic cause of mercury poisoning had not then been diagnosed.

This year, on a weekend, which, as usual in the British National Health Service, meant no functioning microbiology department between Friday 5.00 p.m. and Monday 10.00 a.m., I needed urgent swab and urine samples. After sitting in Casualty for two hours experiencing a lot of pain and great distress, I stormed out with everyone feeling the sharp edge of my tongue. Thinking that this was as good an occasion as any to try out the newly arrived Chinese Herbal Medicine shop in the area, I went there. At 3.00 p.m. on a Saturday afternoon, it was at least open! My symptoms were taken, and I went home with seven packets of a fascinating assortment of barks and plants - all dried of course. The boiling and drinking of the herb broth was unusual; not to be tasted, but downed in one gulp with a mouth rinse of plain water afterwards. It seemed to work reasonably well for the course of the treatment, but there was no lasting relief.

Some years ago my household was introduced to Potters' Peerless Composition Essence herbal remedy traditionally used for alleviation of colds and chills. It contains oak bark, Canadian Pine, poplar bark, prickly ash bark and bayberry bark.

Its effects are instant, and each winter we all had our own bottle at the ready, just in case. It eased the worst of symptoms, and if you caught it in the early stages, then the entire cold or 'flu disappeared. The sting in the tail of it was that it works on an alcoholic basis and it's very sweet. Guess what then added to my influenzae woes? Yes, Thrush!

'Antitis', also from Potters, is good for certain kinds of cystitis. Both these remedies can be in USA health stores.

Because my natural inclination is always to use my own country's health service, I tend to be conventional in my approach to coping with illness. The knowledge I have on cystitis and Candida enables me to prevent them perfectly well. When I knew nothing, of course, I couldn't cope at all. Even though my immune system was so damaged that Candida surged at the drop of a hat, at least I came to know why! And with the removal of all mercury amalgams this threshold has lowered to nothing. I never get Candida now.

I take care to replenish expended energy and know why I feel tired; I can limit chocolate biscuits and not test my damaged immune system overmuch; I refuse Easter egg remnants; I limit and usually refuse wine, sherry or liqueur. In other words, whilst tissue damage remains, I need a personal level of dietary control. This is very comforting in that I can prevent Candidal upsurges myself or deal with a major upsurge if one ever became apparent.

If, through my own negligence, I observe familiar signs then I will certainly use anti-fungal medication as well as withdrawing the obvious causes and resting. Remembering that, before the constant stream of antibiotics for cystitis, I had, to my knowledge, never experienced Candida (perhaps I had in my asthmatic childhood, but if so, it went unnoticed and undiagnosed), my susceptibility subsequently became strong. Amalgam removal has lifted my immune system enormously, hormone levels have declined with menopause as another possible factor and Candida is no threat now.

For those wanting to know what so-called alternative methods offer, I will give a brief run-down. First of all, 'alternative' only means alternative to that provided by conventional doctors in surgeries and hospitals. There is still a false concept about alternative medicine being for cranks and practised by quacks, yet very skilled practitioners of many therapies operate all over the country. Expense can be a problem and it goes without saying that some practitioners are good but lots are not; that many have insufficient qualification or experience and that indeed there are those offering long courses to line their pockets and empty yours! It is best to ask around and to find a multi-functional, well established clinic. There is no doubt, however, that the general public seems willing to try out alternatives locally if their regular doctor is failing them; they also seem prepared to pay the fee and the cost of medications in the hope of a cure, or at least temporary relief.

In terms of Candida counselling, which I offer once this book has been read, tales of rigid diets, costly visits and very costly supplements are frequent. That the victim has come to me from afar and as a last resort, signifies the failure of many alternative practitioners. So I would say to Candida sufferers that conventional science of the body is the firm base from which understanding of Candida begins. It is the reason why I have spent so much time writing the first six chapters. Indisputable medical truths are there. I do not classify myself and my work as any kind of alternative to conventional (i.e. Western) practice or knowledge, because I have neither medical or alternative training. However, it is interesting to find out what is on offer. There is no guarantee that any of them will stop Candida in all sufferers.

Aromatherapy

Essential oils selectively stimulate, revitalise and balance the body's systems. They are widely available in chemists' shops and health food stores. However, aromatherapy and massage is not recommended during any infection and that should include a Candidal upsurge.

WHAT ARE ESSENTIAL OILS?

Essential oils are the aromatic extracts of plants, woods and resins and have been used for thousands of years for medicinal, cosmetic, culinary and domestic purposes. They are wholly natural, complex molecular substances, just as sophisticated as many modern drugs and assist in the normal healing process of the body. They have the ability to influence both body and mind, affecting mood, emotion and physical state. All oils are antiseptic, some more so than others, with Tea Tree having the strongest antiseptic properties. Substitute oils, which smell the same, can be produced synthetically, but do not have the same therapeutic properties. These properties are the result of a reaction of the brain and olfactory systems to stimulation from essential oils. Due to Government legislation, no medicinal claims can be made in respect of essential oils, although they have been used for thousands of years and help a wide variety of conditions.

HOW TO USE ESSENTIAL OILS

Massage

Probably the most pleasurable way to benefit from essential oils is using a maximum of five drops mixed with 10 ml of vegetable carrier oil or base lotion. (To increase or decrease the amount of massage oil, mix half the number of drops to the number of millilitres, e.g. ten drops of essential oil to 20 ml of carrier oil.)

Bath

Add six to eight drops of essential oil to a bath of warm water, mix well and soak for at least ten minutes.

Vaporisation

An ideal way of using aromatherapy in the home. On a fragrancer, add three drops of essential oil to water in the small dish, place over the bulb of a table or standard lamp. Replenish as necessary. Alternatively, use a special oil burner with a small candle.

Inhalations

A bowl of hot water with three drops of essential oils is an effective way to ease breathing problems. Three drops on a tissue is an excellent substitute.

Children

For children under five, use one drop of specified oils; for ages five to fourteen, use half the adult dose.

Neat Lavender may be used on skin for burns, insect bites, etc., but it can cause miscarriages so pregnant women are not advised to use it.

Tea Tree may be used for spots, wounds, etc. These are the only two pure essential oils that may be used in their concentrated form.

Precautions

You should bear the following in mind before using essential oils.

- Use externally only.
- Dilute before use.
- Keep away from children.
- Not to be used without seeking medical advice if pregnant or epileptic.
- Do not exceed the stated dose.
- Keep away from the eyes. Should oil get in the eye, wash thoroughly with cold water for fifteen minutes.

When taking additional homeopathic remedies, check with a practitioner before using essential oils as well. These are all strong and absorbed by skin which then passes them on systemically.

Massage Oils

Grapeseed. Suitable for all types of massage, blends easily with essential oils.
Sunflower and wheatgerm. A blend containing natural vitamin E, which is nourishing for the skin.
Sweet almond. A light oil, used more for facials than a full-body massage.

Base Lotion
Water-based and ideal for localised massage; doesn't mark clothing or leave the skin feeling greasy (use two to three drops of oil in 5 ml of lotion).

Blending
When blending two or more oils together, try to include a top, middle and base note (see below). This gives a longer lasting effect and a pleasant blend.

PURE ESSENTIAL OILS
The following symbols are used to give more information about each oil

M   Suitable for use in massage.
B   Suitable for use in the bath.
V   Suitable for use in a burner or on a light ring.
I   Suitable for inhalation or on a tissue.
C   Suitable for children. Use half the adult dose for children between five and fourteen, and one drop for children under five.
N   May be used neat on the skin for spots, burns, etc.
*   Skin irritation could occur if exposed to strong sunlight or sunbeds. May irritate sensitive skin.
(T)   Top note - aroma lasts up to twenty-four hours.
(M)   Middle note - aroma lasts up to forty-eight hours.
(B)   Base note - aroma lasts up to seven days.

Basil (T)
Stimulating. A digestive aid and excellent mental stimulant, giving the mind strength and clarity. MBVI

Benzoin (B)
Soothing, stimulating. A respiratory aid and calming for all types of skin disorders. MBVI

Bergamot (T)
Uplifting and refreshing. A natural deodorant, relaxing when stressful. Use for cystitis and cold sores. MBVI*

Black Pepper (M)
Warming, soothing. Has a calming effect on stomach upsets. MBVI

Cajeput (T)
Soothing, calming. Mainly used for respiratory and circulatory systems. Excellent used in a vaporiser for colds and flu. A warming oil. MBVI

Caraway (TIM)
A good digestive aid. Excellent for stomach disorders and sleep problems. MBVI

Cedarwood (B)
Soothing. Ideal for oily skin conditions and respiratory problems. MBVI

Camomile (Roman) (M)
Calming, soothing. Commonly used for its anti-inflammatory properties. Benefits sensitive skin and allergies. MBVI

Cinnamon Leaf (MIB)
Powerful. Tooth and gum care, sluggish digestion and stress-related conditions. MBVI

Clary Sage (TIM)
Relaxing and uplifting. Beneficial for female hormonal disorders and pain-relieving during menstruation. Powerful relaxant, said to be euphoric. MBVI

Clove Bud (B)
Uplifting, useful on the gums for toothache. Has a powerful tonic effect on stomach and kidney disorders. MBVI*

Coriander Seed (T)
Stimulating and uplifting. Helpful for digestive problems and warming for arthritic and rheumatic pain. Good mercury chelator. MBVI

Cypress (T)
Balancing, refreshing. Assists with excess perspiration, heavy periods and oily skin. MBVI

Eucalyptus (T)
Soothing, stimulating. Excellent oil for breathing difficulties. Effective for muscular aches and pains. MBVIC

Fennel (M)
Balancing, calming. Maintains body fluid levels, aids digestive disorders. MBVI

Frankincense (B)
Relaxing, soothing. Has ability to slow the breathing, acts as a skin-rejuvenating agent. Used to assist with meditation. MBVI

Geranium (MIB)
Relaxing, refreshing, stimulating. Excellent female oil, regulating the hormonal system. Balances body functions. MBVI

Ginger (M)
Warming, comforting. Aids digestion and muscular aches and pains. Helps to prevent travel sickness. MBVI

Grapefruit (I~
Relaxing, refreshing, uplifting. Used for muscle tone before exercise and muscle fatigue. May assist parasite removal. MBVI*

Hyssop (M)
Soothing for muscular, rheumatic and arthritic pain. **Use with caution. If in doubt, consult a qualified therapist.** MBVI

Jasmine (B)
Relaxing, restoring. King of flowers. Tonic for sensitive skin, helping to restore elasticity. Boosts confidence. MBVI

Juniper (M)
Stimulating, effective for joint mobility, acts as a diuretic, an astringent for acne-prone skin. MBVI

Lavender (M)
Stabilising, relaxing, soothing, calming, uplifting. The most versatile of all the pure essential oils. Balances the body systems. If in doubt, always use lavender except during pregnancy. MBVICN

Lemon (T)
Stimulating, uplifting, refreshing. Effective for poor circulation, used on oily skin. MBVI*

Lemongrass (T)
Soothing, stimulating. Muscular aches and pains benefit from this oil. An effective insect repellent. MBVI*

Lime (T)
Stimulating, uplifting, refreshing. Similar uses to Lemon oil. MBVI*

Mandarin (T)
Soothing, relaxing. Aids digestive disorders, a skin tonic. MBVIC*

Marjoram (M)
Soothing, relaxing, warming. Excellent for joint and muscular aches, soothing for digestive problems, eases pains during the menstrual cycle. MBVI

Melissa Blend (M)
Soothing, uplifting. Non-irritant, suitable for all kinds of allergies. Beneficial for migraine and hayfever sufferers. MBVI*

Myrrh (B)
Soothing. Dilutes to an excellent mouthwash/gargle for sore throats and mouth infections (2% dilution). Gives relief to athlete's foot. MBVI

Neroli (MIB)
Soothing, refreshing, uplifting. Ideal oil for mature sensitive skin, good for thread veins. Boosts the confidence. MBVI

Niaouli (T)
Soothing. Effective on skin eruptions. Makes a good mouthwash/ gargle (2% dilution) for mouth and throat infections. MBVI

Nutmeg (T)
Invigorating. Use with caution, stimulating to nervous system and circulation. Assists the digestive system. MBVI

Orange (T)
Soothing, relaxing, uplifting. Pleasant room freshener. Effective for insomnia. MBVI*

Palmarosa (T)
Uplifting, balancing. Used to regulate sebum production, helpful for stress-related conditions. MBVI

Patchouli (B)
Relaxing, soothing, uplifting. Ideal for chapped or cracked skin, beneficial for fungal infections. MBVI

Peppermint (T)
Cooling, refreshing, uplifting, stimulating. Aids the digestive system, helps clear headaches. MBVI

Petitgrain (TIM)
Relaxing, uplifting. Excellent for stress-related problems, deeply relaxing. MBVI

Pine needle (M)
Refreshing, stimulating. Effective on the respiratory system and helpful for urinary tract infections. MBVI

Rose (B)
Soothing, balancing, tonic. Calming for PMT, excellent for all types of skin care, particularly thread veins. Boosts the confidence. MBVI

Rosemary (M)
Stimulating, uplifting. Exceptionally good for poor circulation, a powerful mental stimulant, balances body fluids. Not to be used by people with high blood pressure. MBVI

Rosewood (M)
Stimulating, good tonic for the skin. Helps the immune system. MBVI

Sage (T)
Seek qualified advice before use.

Sandalwood (B)
Relaxing, soothing. Anti-spasmodic, good for dry coughs, beneficial as mouthwash/gargle for sore throats (2% dilution). A masculine oil. MBVI

Tea Tree (T)
Strong antiseptic. Can be used neat on cuts, bites, etc. Stimulates the immune system. Useful as a household cleanser diluted in rinsing water. MBVIN

Thyme (TIM)
Stimulating. Aids nervous and digestive systems. Very antiseptic. MBVI

Valerian (B)
Sedative, calming. Assists with nervous disorders and insomnia. MBVI

Vertivert (B)
Calming, relaxing. Assists muscular aches and pains and joint mobility. MBVI

Ylang Ylang (B)
Relaxing, uplifting, before sleeping, can slow the heart rate, sensual. Good oil for skin care, ideal to relax before sleeping. MBVI

AROMIX RANGE
These are blends of pure essential oils for specific purposes and should be treated like pure oils, i.e. dilute before use.

Caring range
C1: joint mobility (Cypress, Ginger, Juniper, Marjoram)
C2: after exercise, muscle care (Lavender, Marjoram, Rosemary)
C3: to soothe the head (Lavender, Marjoram, Peppermint)
C4: to relax before sleep (Clary Sage, Lavender, Ylang Ylang)

Feminine range
F1: maintain body fluid balance (Fennel, Geranium, Juniper)
F2: pre-menstrual (Bergamot, Geranium, Rosemary)
F3: excess weight (Fennel, Geranium, Rosemary)
F4: menopause (Cypress, Geranium, Lavender)

Occasion range
O1: easy breathing (Camomile, Frankincense, Lavender)
O2: pollen season (Camomile, Melissa, Lavender)
O3: catarrh and sinus (Cedarwood, Eucalyptus, Pine Needle)

Skincare range
S1: acne-prone skin (Cedarwood, Camomile, Lavender, Lemon-grass)
S2: eczema-prone skin (Camomile, Lavender, Melissa)
S3: psoriasis-prone skin (Bergamot, Camomile, Lavender)
S4: ease lip problems (Bergamot, Eucalyptus, Tea Tree)
S5: ease foot problems (Lavender, Myrrh, Tea Tree)

anti-cellulite (Cypress, Geranium, Juniper)
anti-stretch marks (Frankincense, Lavender, Mandarin)
foot freshener (Cypress, Peppermint)
insect repellent (Eucalyptus, Lavender, Marjoram)
room freshener (Cedarwood, Eucalyptus, Lemon, Orange)

BATH FOAM/SHOWER GELS
New products can be found containing the correct amount of pure essential oil per application for use in the shower.

HAIR CARE
Look for conditioning shampoos covering a variety of uses. Anti-Dandruff, Scalp Tonic, Frequent Wash, Tea Tree, Normal.

LOTIONS
Water-based lotions may have the desired effect by direct application on the skin. Look for:

Acne Lotion	Foot, Freshening Lotion,
After Sun Lotion,	Insect Repellent Lotion,
Anti-Cellulite Lotion,	Lavender Lotion,
Arthritis Lotion,	Moisturising Lotion,
Camomile Lotion,	Rejuvenating Facial Lotion,
Eczema Lotion	Tea Tree Lotion.

There are also many workshops and courses on aromatherapy. Contact your local library for further details. All aromatherapists make up personalised oil requirements for use at home.

Reflexology

This therapy is based on the theory that certain parts of the body reflect the health of major organs. The feet are usually used for diagnosis and then for treatment by variable pressure applied to the appropriate reflex point. This can be done by fingers, thumbs, blunt objects, small balls, rubber bands, clothes pegs or other suitable objects. It is important to consult a qualified and practising reflexologist. Having a go with a friend may be harmful and would be inadvisable even for self-treatment, unless initially guided by the reflexologist.

Once a professional has diagnosed and begun to effect remedial therapy, then reflexology may be used several times a day. Initially, the problem may feel worse, but this is just tenderness in the responding organ. In general, a deep pressure has a tendency to energise.

The feet and hands, whilst being prime areas for reflexology, are not the only ones. Various parts of the mouth, including the tongue, are also very useful especially for problems within the head. Ears also respond well, and Chinese ear acupuncture is another precise form of diagnosis and treatment. For fungal upsurges, try working on:

- feet (for the small intestine, colon areas, adrenal glands, pancreas and thyroid);
- ankles (for the rectum);
- hands (for the small intestines, colon and pancreas)

Ask the reflexologist to diagnose other areas where your energy is weakened and perhaps influencing immune responses. Each side of the body is divided into five zones, ten in total; hands and feet reflect these zones, and in general, the tenderness or pain in treatment pressure is an indication of the extent of the problem within the organ being treated. Understanding these zones is a study in itself. A good reflexologist will have undertaken considerable training.

Acupuncture

This is a really ancient medical practice going back several thousand years. It recognises meridians (lines) of energy which interconnect at dozens of functions (points) all over the body.

When illness occurs, it can be dispersed by feeding or transmitting energy sources to the affected site. By specifically enhancing or redirecting this therapeutic

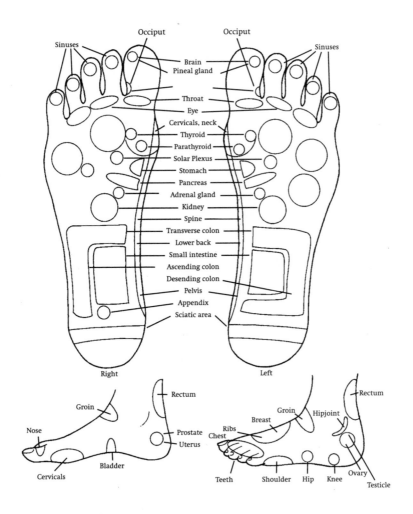

Reflex points on the feet.

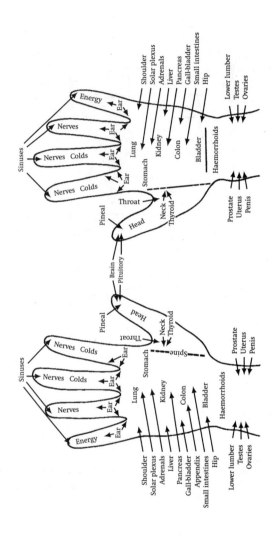

Reflex points on the hands.

energy, the site or organ can be better balanced and able to counteract the illness affecting it. It may be that the energy line is blocked by inflammation and therefore one or more organs along that particular meridian are affected by poor energy flow.

As with all alternative therapies, patients are strongly advised to go to the best practitioner available. It helps to read up a little before an appointment so that you are not 'taken for a ride'.

Since acupuncture involves puncturing the skin with needles, this kind of treatment is not for those who can't stand needles and injections. It also means, of course, that hygiene is of vital importance. Ask about the sterilisation of the needles or make sure that you see the practitioner opening a new pack of needles. It is worth noting that, if you are a blood donor, you are required to inform them before donating, of any acupuncture treatment you have undergone.

Initial diagnosis and many main meridian points commence on each wrist. Pulses indicate any abnormal flows of energy along meridians, and it is a mode of diagnosis in use by many practitioners. Examining the colour, texture and moisture variations of the tongue also reveals a great deal about the state of health. There may be swelling or shrinking of taste buds, cracks, ulcers or fissures; all of these help in firming up a diagnostic picture. Eyes also reflect health and illness. When a small light is shone directly into eyes, the state of clarity, flecks, colours and other marks on the iris will be able to tell a skilled clinician a very great deal.

Most alternative therapists are skilled only within one discipline, and there is a real dearth of doctors who have a grasp on the many different areas which, when combined, provide cheap and effective diagnosis or treatment programmes. India and China, whose centuries-old medicines and treatments have stood the tests of time and usefulness, are perhaps the only true places left where skilled practitioners abound. We, in the West, are very reluctant, because of our own ignorance and suspicion, to place ourselves in the care of a practitioner with whom we have no historical understanding.

Massage

SPINAL THERAPY

In reflexology and acupuncture, there are several sub-therapies combining the main features of reflex and meridians. Since the spine is a major connecting power of the body, spinal therapy and massages, using meridian lines and reflexive pressures,

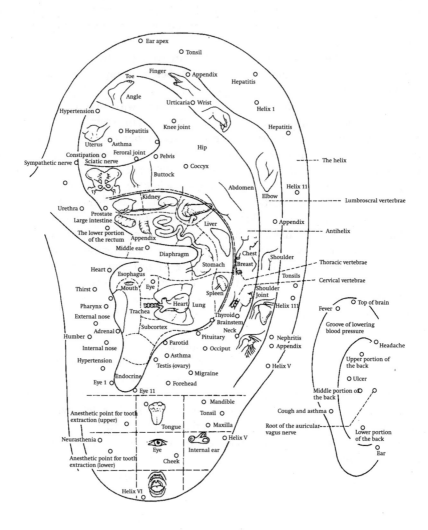

Reflex points on the ears.

can be beneficial. There are four vertebral areas in the spine:

- cervical;
- dorsal;
- lumbar;
- sacral.

Each group of vertebrae encompasses specific areas and organs. Treatment by massaging specific vertebrae or a whole backbone massage is done with oils. Those particularly recommended are cocoa butter, castor oil, peanut oil, olive oil and lanolin.

- For a general massage, use a basic mixture: six parts peanut oil, two parts olive oil, one part lanolin, two parts rosewater and shake the mixture until fully blended.
- For kidney disorders, multiple sclerosis, prostatitis, toxaemia and menopausal problems, mix two parts of olive, two parts peanut oil and one part dissolved lanolin (available from any chemist). For fatigue, glandular disturbances, low vitality, menopausal problems and poor circulation, use peanut oil and a heat lamp overhead.

Again, there is more left out here than can possibly be put in. Find a chiropractor or an osteopath who is registered, qualified and well known. I would add that an osteopath helped cure my childhood asthma, and scepticism about asthma cures from osteopathy are overcome from very well-documented and acceptable research within conventional medicine - just find the best osteopath! No asthma - no steroids - no Candida!

Whilst none of the vertebrae in the list on page 112 specifies fungal infections, they do relate to the glands and organs which feature in fungal upsurges. Most therapies deal with this sort of alliance before looking at any particular symptom; it is the organs and/or their connections that are key to successful diagnosis and treatment.

MASSAGE FOR LYMPH DRAINAGE

We looked earlier at T cells, lymphocytes and such. If blockages occur in the drainage tubes, lymph cannot circulate and cope with wastes. As with blocked arteries causing lethal heart attacks from mercury, toxins and heavy metal storage, so lymph glands, nodes, ducts and flow must be healthy and unobstructed. If

Vertebra	Reflex Area

Cervical (C)

Dorsal (D)

Lumbar (L)

Sacral (S)

C 1 Most parts of the Body
2 Hypothalamus, pituitary, ppineal, eyes. ears, trachea
3 Hypothalamus, face
4 Posterior pituitary, carotid sinus, oesophagus, mouth, nose
5 Shoulders, vocal cords
6 Carotid sinus, Parathyroids, shoulders
7 Posterior pituitary, thymus, carotid sinus, elbows

D 1 Anterior pituitary, thymus, carotid sinus, thyroid, lower arm, oesophagus
2 Bronchials, lungs, vocal cords
3 Heart, Chest
4 Heart
5 Stomach, cardiac & pyloric valves
6 Liver, appendix, diaphragm, pancreas (blood sugar), solar plex
7 Pancreas, gall bladder, splenic flexture, eyes
8 Breast
9 Spleen
10 Ascending & transverse colon, pineal
11 Small intestines, adrenals
12 Kidneys, adrenals, ileocecal valve

L 1 Small intestines sigmoid colon
2 Small intestines, descending colon, hair, skin
3 Gall bladder, adrenals, small intestines, sex organs
4 Kidneys, sigmoid colon, sex glands/organs, sciatica
5 Kidneys, adernals, urethra, legs

Sacral
Hip bones, buttocks
rectum, anus

Reflex points on the spine.

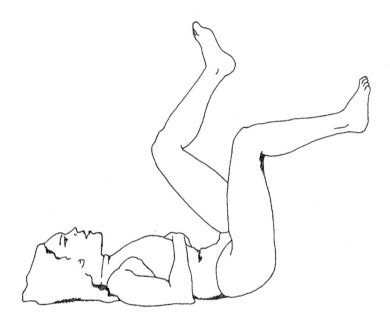

Exercise to improve lymph circulation, take care if you suffer back problems.

wastes build up, bacterial/yeast balance can be affected.

It is possible to use massage to keep lymph running freely and clear obstructions usually caused by inflammation, infections and systemic illnesses. Most practitioners understand the lymph system and can undertake specific lymph massaging. Once the process is understood, try it at home. To drain all the lymph tissues in the trunk of the body, lie on your back and bicycle in the air, either with your trunk flat or balancing more on your shoulders, supporting hips with hands. This clears the pelvic region, groin, digestive system, pancreas, liver and kidneys. It should always be preceded by a massage of the lymph glands either side of the neck using light, circular movements.

MASSAGE FOR DIGESTION (ENERGY)

This was originally researched by the Boyeson family and seems a very sensible way to encourage peristalsis (the muscular contractions that move food down through the large/small intestine). A quicker digestion, collection or absorption of body nutrients and final rejection of wastes, including excess bacteria and yeasts, can only be very beneficial to sufferers from Candida upsurges.

The Boyesons argued that pent-up emotions go sour. Misdirected and accumulated emotional energy unbalances energy distribution. This is then reflected in the intestines; if you are excited or have a good emotional balance, there is an increase in peristaltic waving helping to propel wastes and keep the intestines cleared. If the emotional balance is negative and lethargic or if antibiotics/drugs have slowed digestion, peristalsis declines.

The sounds of our intestines can indicate their condition, as Candida sufferers know only too well. Magnified by a stethoscope, these sounds can be thunderous! They should be placid, like a quiet stream, with a flattened abdomen indicating no faecal build-up and, therefore, a daily bowel movement.

Massage movements are smooth and have to be undertaken by a trained practitioner whose job it is to find outlets for these pent-up emotions. Strokes always go from the middle to outer edges of the body. The misdirected energy is now sent in several directions and to several places. Wrists, neck, waist, joints, ankles, eye sockets, nose, chin, shoulders and ribs are the main areas for effective release.

All of us are familiar with the tensions brought on by office politics, jobs, relationships and general day-to-day aggravations. Bowels are always better for a good walk or an exciting challenge of some sort like singing a difficult solo. Holidays can produce better peristalsis - better psycho-energy release, the Boyesons might argue.

Energy

Energy dispersal by digestive massage is pertinent to understanding a little more about energy itself. From the chapter on glucose production and control, we know that all foods, particularly carbohydrates and sugars, end up as alcohol and carbon dioxide. This alcohol from nutritional sources is only one form of energy gathering done by the body. Now we have just touched upon another - emotional/brain energy, that is, the incoming data from around us collated and presented in the brain, which makes us feel balanced or excited or depressed and many levels in between. It's worth having a quick look at other energy sources.

SUNLIGHT

As with all plant life, human and animal life can also derive energy from sunshine. Not only is it taken in by direct outside contact, but it can be fed back in nutritional sources. The yellow/orange/red colour of all sun-ripened fruits and vegetables occurs because they have absorbed sunlight. In moderation, body energy lowered by intestinal imbalance may acquire extra vitamins and energy colours through bright fruits and vegetables. Vitamins from these sources are also helpful, as discussed earlier in the book; most commonly found are A, Bs and E.

Five to ten minutes' exposure every day when the sun is out, whether spring, summer, autumn or winter, helps boost energy supplies. It must be the pure thing - no windows or glasses between yourself and the sun, it shouldn't be midday summer sunshine and, when possible, the whole body should be exposed. But don't overdo it. Over-exposure is ageing, cancer-forming and tiring.

ELECTRICITY

We all know about electrical storms.

After one electrical storm in London, not only were police and fire services inundated, but so were hospital casualty units, paramedics and local doctors; oxygen supplies were swiftly depleted as a result of the increase in asthma and tightened breathing cases. We are used to a natural earth surface with negative electrical charges creating only minor voltage changes, but the passionate charging of an electrical storm has noticeable effects.

A direct current, DC, charge from an electric shock, or indeed a lightning strike, disrupts electrical body systems, causing pain, tingling, shock, variable paralysis or even death. We, as humans and as creatures of earth, are electrically energised. Too much or too little additional electricity affects our wellbeing.

In normal conditions, the higher you climb up a mountain, the greater the current, especially if there is no moisture in the air; conversely, in low, marshy, damp areas voltage is reduced. In an electrical storm, harmful positive lightning charges are overwhelmingly high, since they originate in the ionosphere and flash voltage down to us. As the currents of the earth are extremely low, it is the abrupt changes which create health reactions. Any metals on, or surrounding, a house or office may cause counter-electricity fields which deplete normal earth energy.

Plastics and synthetics, in offices particularly, may begin to explain some of the 'sick building syndrome', especially with all the strong electric fields created by office equipment like computers, typewriters, photocopiers, boilers, power lines and much more. Absence of fresh air compounds the field and, for the working day of six hours or more, can create poor health and energy. To combat this, go for a stroll at lunchtime, ask for at least one window to be open and eat a good lunch without alcohol.

Household appliances and power tools, televisions, electric fires or blankets, mobile phones, sub-stations or overhead wires near the home may also drain human energy, resulting in immuno-suppression and constant poor health. This is perhaps a new concept to many of us, but the healthy use of energy sources is paramount in the battle to help maintain intestinal balance and a healthy immune system. Mercury fillings and gold caps also create oral electrical currents .

CLOTHING AND HOUSING

It is a good general rule that natural fibres and materials allow static and stored body electricity to disperse from us and from our environment. Clothes should be cottons, linens, silks, wool. Rayon seems to be the only man-made material which does not charge so strongly. Nylon, as in tights, stockings, underwear, etc., should be avoided. Bright colours balance a grey day or mood, and black and grey should be worn rarely. Leather soles on shoes promote an outward release of electricity from legs and feet. Going barefoot at home for a few minutes can help considerably.

Large blocks of flats with metal-reinforced concrete create static electric traps for the humans inside. Vulnerable, energy-depleted people need to live in brick, wood, stone or fibrocement and avoid copper, lead or plastic piping (galvanised iron or ceramic is best). Internal decoration is best left as brick or stone walls; walk on wooden floors with rugs; avoid paint and metals; have cotton or linen curtains; try cooking two days meals in one session; instal solar panels for natural heating supplies.

The list can go on, but I think that this is enough to draw attention back, when possible, to using natural sources to enhance personal and environmental clean living. The basic message is that fresh air and sunlight are good for us. These are essentially anti-fungal, being the opposite of dark and moist.

Homeopathy

Homeopathy could be said to be based on the principle of vaccination discussed earlier; that is by using a tiny amount of the bacteria/spores/mucus harvested from the particular disease, e.g. polio, antibodies can be artificially introduced in a healthy person. This protects against a possible future attack by having an appropriate defence response ready. Homeopathy, too, is based on the concept of treating like with like. By great distillation and dilution, tiny amounts of the toxin are introduced to combat the ailment. Remedies are ancient, well tested and made from an array of plants, minerals, animals or chemicals. Usually, the remedy is taken as pillules under the tongue or by droplets from a small phial. Pillules are sugar-coated, though, and not recommended for diabetics or yeast sufferers.

A qualified, registered homeopathic practitioner in your area may have some worthwhile ideas for improving any health problems causing a depressed immune system. Listen to their views on fungal treatment, and if they understand or coincide with the basic truths of fungal infestation, then consider treatment. Beware of any suggestions of rigid diets since these cannot be implemented forever and they reduce general energy and wellbeing, leaving a further weakened immune system.

Herbal medicines

Herbal medicines are medicines made from parts of plants, e.g. roots, flowers, barks, or extracts from them. For example, Senna leaf and Senna pods are well-known laxatives. And because herbal medicines are totally natural being environmentally friendly, they do not pollute the planet and they consume less of our limited energy resources. European law now enshrines herbal medicine as making a proven and viable contribution to Europe's health care.

It is one of the oldest known forms of medicine - there are examples recorded in the earliest records, from the Dead Sea Scrolls to the Pyramids, mentioning the use of herbs as medicines. There is even evidence that cavemen used certain plants which were obviously not for their food value and are thought to have been used as medicines.

Herbal medicines should not be confused with homeopathic remedies. They are not diluted, as is the case with homeopathic medicines (often one part per million, or less). Herbal medicines work by stimulating the body to cure itself but homeopathic medicines use many herbs, minerals and animal extracts as required.

The effectiveness of herbal medicines is well documented. Man has observed for hundreds of years that herbs have an obvious and easily measured effect, from the first day dock leaves were rubbed onto nettle stings, to the now well-known use of foxglove as a major heart drug. In fact, over sixty per cent of the world's population has no other kind of medicine but herbal available to them. Billions of people and millions of doctors from China to the Americas have researched and observed the effectiveness of these herbs.

The herbal practitioners, who devised the formulas after years of experience with patients, took a holistic view of treatment. Holistic medicine treats the whole person and provides pharmacologically active remedies for each of the body systems. With most illnesses, there is usually a major cause and a variety of different symptoms. By treating all the aspects of the ailment with different herbs, the patient often feels a rapid improvement.

TAKING HERBAL MEDICINE

Herbal medicines are softer and gentler than chemical drugs, and their effects are more gradual, but longer lasting. If they are to work well, a steady stream of the herb is essential, which is why it is usually necessary to take a herbal remedy three or four times a day and over a reasonable period of time, such as four weeks. The remedy should be taken for as long as symptoms persist or for the prescribed duration of the course. Gentler remedies often require longer use, and you should continue until improvement arrives. You must also be patient and not be tempted to increase the dose to achieve quicker results. The dosage has been set by experts, and this should be followed carefully. Remember that herbal medicines work differently from chemical drugs, and whereas you can often see very quick results with the latter just by taking two pills a day, it can take several weeks for the effect of herbal remedies to become apparent.

Herbal medicines can be used to treat an enormous variety of complaints, including seemingly incurable problems like arthritis. It's unfortunate that, for many, herbal medicine is a last resort, which is perhaps why it often has such a striking effect - people still don't expect it to work. Deciding which product to take usually depends on the nature of the complaint. If it's a simple disease, like a cough or cold or a digestive, nervous, rheumatic or functional problem, you can usually pick out a product yourself by reading the label. For more serious complaints, visit a practitioner first for diagnosis. You can then select the medicine of your choice, whether herbal or chemical. If, however, the symptoms persist, consult your practitioner again.

It is usually possible to take two or more herbal medicines for different problems at the same time. For simple complaints, such as a cough and a sore throat, there are no known side-effects of doing this. If in doubt, consult your practitioner or pharmacist.

If you are also on a prescription for chemical drugs, you should tell your doctor you are planning to take any other medication including herbal - even if it's only indigestion tablets. Often they may be taken together, but each needs separate evaluation.

Herbal medicines can usually be given safely to children, but always read the label carefully, as the dosage may be different. Don't give any medicines to children under five without consulting your practitioner. There is more of a difference of opinion when it comes to women who are pregnant or breast-feeding. General advice is always to take no medicine at all, but do consult your practitioner, as gentler remedies may be allowed. If you are vegetarian or vegan, check with your retailer that the medicine you have chosen is suitable. Herbal medicines have very few known side-effects. Licensed herbal medicines with a Product Licence have been vetted for all aspects of safety. Nor are herbal medicines addictive, as proven by years of clinical experience. This is one reason why there has been a substantial growth in herbal medicines, particularly in the area of herbs for relaxation and sleeping.

However, as with any medication, if you experience any strange feelings or effects, you are advised to stop and consult your practitioner. Remember also that, like most medicines, herbal medicines have a limited shelf life, and this should be marked on the label. Herbal medicines should be stored in a cool place with the lid firmly closed and out of the reach of children. Dispose of out-of-date medicines carefully or take them to a pharmacy or health-food shop.

PRODUCTION OF HERBAL MEDICINES

Even as late as the 1950s, the majority of pharmaceutical products were herbal or herbal-based. Since then, there has been an explosion in the use of chemicals in drugs, mainly for serious disorders, that has eclipsed the older herbal medicines. Many unwanted contra-indications are listed on Western medications and patients are becoming more interested in herbal remedies. The new European standard of licensing has given pharmacists the confidence to carry a limited range of herbal products, while health-food and specialist shops carry a wide range. In mainland Europe, herbal drugs are in common use in general health care and most mainstream medicines have origins in plant or animal substances. Back in the late 1960s, after the problem with thalidomide, the UK government passed a very exacting law, the 1968 Medicines Act, which required all medicines, including licensed herbal remedies, to be made in a factory with a Manufacturer's Licence (ML). This governs every aspect of manufacture and quality control and means that the factory is regularly inspected by Department of Health officials. Even more importantly, in the run-up to the Single European Market, there was a review of all medicines, including herbal, and the Product Licence (PL) was introduced. In order to have a Product Licence on the pack, the manufacturer has had to satisfy Department of Health doctors that each herbal medicine is safe, pure and effective. Under the terms of the Product Licence, manufacturers have to carry out exacting surveys to control any possible contamination from fertilisers, pesticides, etc. All such standards must be met before the quality-control laboratory can release a product for sale. The presence of the Product Licence or Manufacturer's Licence is your guarantee that the product has been properly tested and assessed and the claims on the pack are proven. In addition, the product review in 1991, plus new European standards, lifted the level of science to a new high. Scientific standards and methods are always applied to herbal medicines where appropriate. The herbs in all medicines are under constant review and if any problems were to occur, the product would be immediately removed from the market. These two Licences are your guarantee of a safe remedy.

Herbal medicines are generally cheaper than other remedies, although their cost has increased somewhat in recent years. New European legislation has demanded even more exacting tests and controls, all introduced in 1991 when herbal medicines gained full recognition as mainstream medicine. Licensed herbal products have to display a guaranteed shelf life which is achieved by wrapping them in a natural sugar coating often coloured with natural dyes for ease of identification.

Minerals and vitamins

This is an area of interest to many alternative practitioners of all disciplines. Continuous courses of supplements are costly so be sure that you need them. Clearly, a sensible diet of three meals a day should contain compounds of primary nutrients, and any advice to take supplements should recognise that. However, allergic people particularly are less able to absorb nutrients, and those struggling with poor health and depleted immunity may well require additional sources. Soil is overworked and denuded of naturally occurring minerals and vitamins. Family life with several people in one household and a skilled Mother cooking wholesome food has become a luxury. Many 'households' are singles, not good at cooking. Lots more alcohol in the diet strains kidneys and liver and depletes mineral levels. It is also true that mercury swallowed or inhaled from teeth fillings depletes Magnesium, Calcium and Manganese on a permanent basis until safe removal is undertaken.

Here are some minerals and vitamins that may be useful for sufferers of Candida:

- Blurred vision: vitamins B2, B6, pantothenic acid.
- Dry skin: vitamins A, C, Essential Fatty Acids (EFAs) (linoleic and linolenic, as found in ground-linseed oil, cod-liver oil and evening primrose oil).
- Eczema and ulcers of all sorts: vitamins C, B2, B6, niacin, EFAs, zinc, magnesium.
- Fungal infestations of skin: B vitamins, localised packs or baths of Epsom salts.
- Itching skin: B vitamins, C, EFAs.
- Inflamed, pus-head spots: vitamin B6, zinc.
- Blackened skin: vitamins C, B2 bioflavonoids.
- Vaginal itching: vitamins B2, E, C.
- Urticaria: vitamins B6, C, zinc.
- White, brittle, infected nails: zinc, vitamin B6.
- Peeling nails: vitamins A, C, calcium.
- Ridged nails: vitamin A, more protein.
- Scaling of nails: biotin.
- Enlarged tongue: pantothenic acid.
- Burning, sore tongue: vitamins B2, B6, B12, niacin.
- Cracked lips and corners of mouth: vitamins B2, B6, folic acid.
- Furrowed tongue: vitamin B1, pantothenic acid.
- Mouth ulcers: folic acid, vitamin B6, zinc.
- Enlarged taste buds: niacin/nicotinamide.
- Sore, inflamed tongue: niacin, vitamin B6.
- White patches on tongue: vitamin B2, other B vitamins.

If the tongue is white, there is intestinal putrefaction; if it is yellowish or brown, then liver or gall-bladder problems should be investigated.

Regular doses of magnesium, zinc, calcium, chromium, manganese, potassium, selenium, sulphur, molybdenum, iron, iodine may be helpful to people with an allergic/fungal predisposition. We need all these to promote a healthy immune system. Vitamins should include A, B1 (thiamin), B2 (riboflavin), B6 (pyridoxine), B12, C, D, E. Acids should include folic, nicotinic, pantothenic, pangamic, inositol.

NUTRITIONAL ACID/ALKALINE LEVELS

Malfunctioning digestive enzymes causing poor digestion and therefore affecting breakdown of food, absorption of nutrients and dispersal of glucose may be helped by careful supplementing of the following: pancreatin, papain, bromelain, pepsin, bile, hydrochloric acid, lemon juice, ascorbic acid. These come in tablets to be swallowed whole. A low maintenance dose may be taken of pancreatin with a combination tablet consisting of bile, pepsin, papain and bromelain.

Where gastric acid levels are dropping because of degenerative disease or old age, there are tablets of hydrochloric acid and pepsin which can be taken during high-protein meals where extra help with protein digestion is required. Where food is uncooked, enzyme supplement is not required. Any enzyme supplements should be taken *during* a meal. Practitioner guidance is suggested.

An approximate guideline for acidity/alkalinity levels relating to pancreatic enzymes is as follows: litmus paper showing blue when pressed into the roof of the mouth influenced by saliva will prove alkalinity; red proves acid and a lilac colour shows neutral. Modern indicator papers are more precise; ask the pharmacist which he would recommend. The pH of saliva is normally 6.4 to 6.8 before a meal, but thirty minutes after a protein meal it should increase to above 6.8. This is caused by the stomach lining producing alkaline mucus to protect itself against rising gastric-juice production to help break down the food. If the pH does not rise above 6.8, the stomach remains too acidic for pancreatic enzymes and hormones to fully activate within the digestive process. One quarter of a level teaspoon of bicarbonate of soda may be taken after an hour or so to encourage the enzymes. If the pH level zooms above 6.8 or remains at the pre-meal level (i.e. only slightly acidic), then reactions in the stomach are insufficiently acid and the tablet containing hydrochloric acid and peptin taken with subsequent meals may be helpful. Ascorbic acid (vitamin C) or lemon juice will also be helpful.

Timing meals

Water should not be drunk during a meal, since it dilutes the acidity required for better digestion. Preferably, drink a glass of water beforehand. Drinking water is most effective before breakfast to cleanse and prepare the digestive tract after several hours of stagnation. Carbonated water is not recommended, despite its popularity, since it is full of carbon dioxide and alkaline substances.

The stomach needs to be acid for quick food breakdown. You should have a good breakfast to maintain energy levels until lunchtime and to conserve the energy renewal and energy formation brought about during sleep. Lunch should be nutritious and provide another big energy boost to combat exercise, effects of travel, housework, stress, etc., which burn off sleep and breakfast resources constantly during the day. The evening meal should not be taken after 8.00 p.m. and should preferably be over by 7.30 p.m. so that the sleep cycle can begin with all food well past the stomach and large intestine. Daybreak and nightfall are the timed cycles which begin and end the digestive body clock. Electric light stopped all that!

Food combining.

Some experts believe that combining protein and starches may be detrimental to digestion. Protein meals require high levels of gastric juice, and even within proteins, there are different gastric juice requirements. Proper digestion of starches (carbohydrates) is aided by enzyme activators such as the B vitamins, chloride, calcium and magnesium. A basic guide to food combination is as follows:

- Don't eat meat, fish, eggs, dairy products, nuts or oils together.
- Don't eat apples, melons (i.e. quick-fermenting fruits) and fruit juices with other foods.
- Don't put milk in tea or coffee, and cut back on your intake of these anyway.

As an alternative, try one of the many delicious herb teas now available in supermarket. Peppermint or Camomile tea are amongst many which can be taken in small amounts after meals.

Contemplating all this apparently thoroughly sound and reasoned advice contrasts strongly with common dietary habits. I can quote countless examples, as I'm sure everyone could, of flagrant violations of these simple guidelines which might help poor digestion and discourage the conditions which promote Candidal upsurges. It would take very radical changes in shopping, preparation of menus and mealtimes to alter current habits. Nevertheless, the base site, our digestive system, is where Candida upsurges commence.

In updating this book I am mindful all the time of mercury's influence on digestion. Irritable Bowel Syndrome (IBS), Crohn's Disease, Inflammatory Bowel disorders are all in the anti-mercury literature. For myself, all my life until amalgam removal one mouthful of food would cause pain. When substantial gas or pain halted eating I was distressed but there seemed no answer and unless the pain was excruciating I thought it all normal! It wasn't. With safe amalgam removal, eating soon became pain-free, it was nothing short of miraculous. Bowels started acting on a daily basis with a well-formed stool. Wind, pain, belching, constipation, faecal smell, straining, swollen haemorrhoids from childbirth all changed with time and some re-training. I am furious that my body has been so stressed since I was little because of what dentists have put into me.

LAXATIVES

Anything helping good daily or twice daily expulsion of faecal waste is important because toxinous bacterial build-up is thwarted and much ill health prevented. If faecal back-up in the colon slows peristalsis in the intestines, then there is more work for the kidneys in sifting excessive wastes.

This is equally true for those whose Candida levels appear to be high for any of the reasons already discussed and those still to come. It is not acceptable to sit back and do nothing about constipation. If all else is failing to make bowels work, organize safe amalgam removal.

Nowhere can you read of what a normal bowel movement should be like. It should start with feeling of movement or 'excitement' somewhere behind the bladder towards the back. Find a toilet as soon as possible, quickly, because if you 'deny' it, more convenient expulsion later may involve straining. If away from home, line the seat with tissue paper and sit comfortably. The moving stool can be felt coming down either into the bowel or from the intestine into it. As it begins to emerge sit fairly straight, even lean back but don't bend forward at this point to strain, let the strong muscles do their job and the stool should be one longish line of waste material. I can always remember being immensely impressed at a Beirut hostage's comment that since his mother had trained his bowels from childhood to work every day at 7.00am, he always knew, though imprisoned in the dark 24 hours a day for two years, that another day had started!

Of course, illness, lack of exercise, meats, too much flour, pasta or rice will harden the stool so drink water to help counteract this. Fibrous fruits and husks can all help to keep stool formation softer and easier to pass just like animal dung. Urgent bowel movements can start from fear, excitement, food poisoning, too much coffee or caffeine, climate changes and many personal inconvenient variations!

Ideas for relieving constipation.

Oat bran
Taken each morning in semi-skimmed milk with no sugar. It may occasionally include wheat bran, but this tends to clog the ridged walls of the intestines, and too much will actually cause constipation.

Epsom salts
Taken mixed with water.

Syrup of figs
This is an old laxative, but sugary, so Candida sufferers may want to avoid this one.

Mustard seeds

Taken with a garlic capsule. Mix half a teaspoon of dried seeds with water and drink twice daily before meals. This reduces gases in the intestines and improves bowel action. Stop if it has adverse effects, and don't try it if you have a history of upset stomachs or irritable bowels.

Prunes

These aren't good for people with insecure blood sugar levels, but otherwise they are a good natural laxative.

Senna pods

These are the basis of many laxatives.

Water

This is a good stomach cleanser when taken before breakfast.

The greatest aid to a regular bowel is to withdraw refined white sugar and refined white flour/rice from the diet. Laxatives will still have to 'struggle against the tide' if anti-peristaltic food is still being eaten. It is better to take a gentle laxative three times a week and have regular bowel movements than to strain and struggle. If your body becomes used to one kind of laxative, change or rotate those suiting you best.

Summary

No one can be expected to alter their daily life so radically that they become a misery to themselves and to other people. This chapter has simply sought to draw attention to additional possibilities for enhancing the immune system and helping remove fungal levels at all possible points. There are many alternative health disciplines and opportunities, but by cost alone they are often self-limiting and often too rigorous to maintain for ever. Always look for a qualified or registered practitioner in the district and ask around for any comments from previous clients.

A good, general, daily supplement of minerals and vitamins, or just those in which you are deficient, may go a long way to help stabilise an unstable immune system. Immunity will fluctuate - but when we are trying to limit or stop Candidal upsurge, we must at least preserve the base site activities - those in the digestive system. Achieving that intimate balance between bacteria and yeasts is an inter-dependent circle of nutrition, exercise, energy, treatment and other self-help, which we are now going to add to all that has gone before.

Removing mercury amalgam safely and considering effects of other dental metals present in your mouth can completely change the way your bowels work. The competing and constant territorial war between bacteria and fungi in the gut is also harmonized by safe mercury amalgam removal. Your own dentist will probably not be able to help, only those well-trained in safe removal can. Interview those in your area!

9 Orthodox treatments

As we have seen so far, there can be no doubt from medical research and proof, that Candida Albicans is a common condition. It can be found in any area of the body, both external and internal, but is more prevalent in warm, dark, moist areas together with a good supply of sugary, yeasty nutrition. It prefers a weakened immune system, a fact that no doctor should deny. Whilst tests are sometimes negative, greater reliance should be placed on past history and any previously positive tests. When newer tests become more reliable, the situation will improve.

Getting a positive test

The conditions under which tests are taken count considerably in achieving a 'positive' result. For instance, ear swabs will prove negative if the ear canal is dry. It needs to be wet or discharging for the cotton-wool swab to accumulate organisms. A cleaned-out vagina will be very unlikely to show thrush or anything else, so don't clean it out if you know you're going to have a swab.

If there is systemic Candida to be proved, first make the case for this possibility in writing, together with symptoms, and do not attempt any treatment by mouth or by self-help. Self help at this stage may reduce lab chances of a correct diagnosis.

Proof goes a long way to gaining credence at the health centre. That miserable feeling of not being taken seriously by the doctor is a mountain common to all Candida sufferers. Proving your case can entail careful timing. If the surgery works to appointments, this may mean hanging on - you will not gain credence by using emergency facilities for thrush of the finger nails! Conversely, a vaginal emergency is often best dealt with at the Emergency Room or Genito Urinary department of the nearest large hospital, so always make sure you have its number and hours somewhere safe.

Remember that between 7.30 p.m. on a Friday and 11.30 a.m. on a Monday, the microbiology department is closed to outside sampling from surgeries. This means that swabs and samples are not delivered to the laboratory, but are kept somewhere else. By Monday morning, the samples are highly unlikely to be dependable.

Organisms will have declined due to lack of nutrition. Always take a sample correctly if you have to do one at home, promptly attend any appointment for professional sample-taking and be prepared for some Candida samples to be taken in hospital itself.

If you are already seriously ill in hospital and either you, a relative, doctor or nurse thinks that Candida is present, ask for tests and treatment. A friend of mine eased his dying father's final weeks by knowing about systemic Candida. His father was having great difficulty in swallowing because his tongue was swollen and his mouth and throat very dry. A nurse was asked whether she felt this was Candida. Without this prompting, no action would have been taken. Sucking an anti-fungal lozenge relieved much discomfort.

Do not be too dismayed if test results show negative. Anything could have happened to the sample taking, or the sample delivery, or the sample culturing. If you are absolutely sure that this is a return of the old enemy, then pursue it! Faced with this knowledge, the doctor may be 'persuaded' or inclined to write a prescription; there is all the self-help, too.

Pharmaceutical medications

At present the annual growth rate of anti-fungal medications in the world market is running at nineteen per cent. Turnover increased by from £1.6 billion at 1993 levels to over £3 billion by 1997, an enormous reflection of the continuously rising incidence of fungal infections. This does not only represent Candida Albicans, but also its sub-strains and Aspergillus, which is a nasty lung fungus. Organisms responsible for athlete's foot and ringworm are included in these figures.

Amphotericin B was the chief systemic treatment on prescription until 1990, when Diflucan, from Pfizer, came onto the market. This has proved variable in its help; as a replacement for Amphotericin B, it overcame the earlier side-effects of that drug and represented a great advance; however, the one-day dose which was so highly lauded does not have lasting results. For simple vaginal thrush in new patients, it did well enough, but not as a treatment for more ingrained Candida at the vaginal site. As a single dose for systemic Candidosis, it has not done the job. If Diflucan is to be prescribed, it must be done so over longer courses. Diflucan does not work against a broad spectrum of fungi, and there are also increasing cases of resistant Candida. Pfizer is researching to amend these difficulties. Amphotericin B is similarly being reformulated to reduce side-effects and potency.

Nizoral from Johnson & Johnson carries a warning about liver deterioration, and blood tests for liver function are recommended after a course. This does not make it a popular choice either for doctors or patients, since more effort and costs are involved.

Sporanox by Janssen Pharmaceuticals is expensive, but active against all known fungi, not just Candida. It can be prescribed for anywhere between seven and twenty-eight days. The longer therapy of two or three weeks in severe, systemic Candida is best so that any deep-seated spores or reproduction cycles can also be eradicated. It is, in my opinion, the best systemic preparation currently available. As with many drugs, Sporanox is not to be taken by pregnant women.

Sporanox is derived from itraconazole, Diflucan comes from fluconazole and Nizoral from ketoconazole. All three are only available on prescription and are chemically manufactured from a group called 'azoles'; other brand names and generic azoles are:

- Canestan (clotrimazole);
- Microspore (bisonazole);
- Lotrisone (clotrimazole);
- Daktarin/Monistat (miconazole).

As well as azoles, other sources of anti-fungal medications are on trial, undergoing licensing or research. They include Ambisome by Vestar Pharmaceuticals and Amphocil by Liposome (known as Zeneca outside North America and Japan), and are both recommended for use with very severe systemic Candida where other drugs have failed.

Of drugs that are not azole-based, Lamisil from the Swiss firm, Sandoz, deals well with skin Candida at all body sites. Lamisil is the market leader of skin Candida preparations and actually kills the fungus. There are future possibilities for its systemic use.

All the azole-based drugs interfere with fungal cell membranes, thus controlling their upsurge; they are fungistatic. Lamisol and other non-azole drugs kill the fungi and are called fungicidal. Around the world fungal infections are big news, with vast sums being spent on new compounds to meet this surging demand.

PRESCRIBABLE DRUGS

For systemic candida

Sporanox, Diflucan, Miconazole, Flucytosine, Amphoteracin B, Immune26.

For intestinal sites only (no systemic value)
Nystatin.

For ears
Gentisone drops (Gentisone HC helps itching), Canestan drops, Econazole (lotion or cream). I personally found Betnovate cream (orange label) extremely good when sparsely smeared into the ear; this stopped my long-term Candidal ear infection but doctors would laugh at this. Also systemic drugs.

For eyes
Gentisone eye/ear drops, Cidomycin eye/ear drops, Sporanox and other systemics.

For mouth and tongue
Nystatin pastilles, Daktarin oral gel (**OTC**), Fungilin lozenge.

For all skin sites
Lamisil, Mucospor, Ecostatin, Pevaryl, Nizoral, Dermonistat, Trosyd, Sulconazole, as creams. Systemics may also be appropriate.

For thrush of vagina and penis
Sporanox or Diflucan (short oral dose), Gynodaktarin pessaries and cream, Terazol cream/pessary, Candeptin cream, Nystatin cream/ pessaries, Canestan (**OTC**) pessary (one pessary), Monistat/Pevaryl/ Canestan creams, Femeron (**OTC**) pessary (one pessary).

For scalp yeasts
Nizoral shampoo. Polytar shampoo morning and night. Herbal products.

For oesophageal thrush
Systemics, gels or lozenges. But stop the steroid inhaler since it is the main cause.

For immuno-compromised, severely ill patients, intravenous drips of flucytosine may be recommended; Sporanox may be prescribed for longer periods, and Diflucan can also be administered by intravenous drip.

All these drugs are prescribable. The doctor should check in MIMMS directory of drugs and conditions for appropriate doses, contraindications and any other drug reactions with those already being taken. This section only seeks to name some of the available choices because new products come to market regularly. The usual rules for pregnancy, liver, heart, kidney observations and discussions with doctors must always apply.

In the USA, vaginal creams and tablets are available over the counter without prescription. Monistat and Gyne-Lotrimin are advertising in women's magazines, to great effect upon everyone's purses; doctors are by-passed, frustration avoided and sales surge. In Britain, we only have two medications available over the counter: Canestan and Femeron but, doubtless, more will follow. Elsewhere in the world, all these anti-fungal medications are instantly available over the counter. New drugs come regularly to market so discuss latest additions to the anti-fungal range.

Desensitisation

In chapter 6, we looked at the immune system, allergies, innoculations and vaccinations. Not everyone accepts deep intra-muscular vaccination against diseases such as tuberculosis, diphtheria and others. Many research programmes around the world are looking again at vaccination possibilities for problems such a Thrush or E.Coli infections but it cannot be a good thing in harmony with Nature to keep introducing viruses to the human body. Modern vaccine materials contain preservatives, anti-bacterials and a range of animal viruses including 40 kinds from monkeys. This is a step too far.

In Britain and the USA, there are conventionally trained doctors who, because they have been unable to accept the constraints of conventional practice, have branched out into setting up their own private clinics. Ahead of their peers, yet firmly rooted in fact and research, they practise desensitisation against Candida and general yeasts and moulds. Obviously full assessments and tests have been carried out before treatment.

Asthma and allergy desensitisation on the State has fallen into an abyss elsewhere because a few patients, improperly and impersonally treated, had acute reactions; as a result, there are millions using steroids, beta-blockers or inhalers who may not need to use these very doubtful forms of long-term treatment.

EPD allergy injections are administered just underneath the skin, not deep, nor into blood vessels. They contain the purest and freshest materials. No viruses, antiseptics or additives are used. This treatment is called EPD- Enzyme Potentiated Desensitisation.

Any long-term treatment like Beta-blockers causing side effects cannot be the best treatment. Desensitisation may be a better answer. EPD is far more effective in terms of costs, fewer side effects, improved treatment and illness relief. This kind of therapy may be well suited for people with an underlying weakened immune system from past attacks, illnesses, accidents or bad health; it may also help those who inherited a genetic malfunction, causing a quickened response to Candida, moulds or fungal upsurge. Case-history-taking is probably the best way of deciding such factors, since immunologists are perhaps rather fanciful specialists in the eyes of the general practitioner. You can always try asking for a referral to one!

EPD, Enzyme Potentiated Desensitisation deals with the enzymes which encourage Candidal strength. It also understands a wide range of allergies, such as foods, chemicals or environmental, discovered in the case-history-take. One tiny injection can deal with the lot and, again, I speak with great personal knowledge and authority. My own acute, multi-allergic body began this treatment in 1982 in London with Dr Len McEwen. Except in the heaviest hayfever time, I lost my shocking allergic rhinitis. It went gradually in eighteen treatments over eight years. For some years this wonderful treatment kept me sane but then, we think, the dental anaesthetics used in quantity for removing all the mercury amalgam and four gold caps affected the EPD protection. Dental treatment is not advised four weeks before or after EPD injections. I have had to start all over again and am well whilst the injection protection lasts. It becomes apparent to about three weeks notification that I need the next one. Individual patients have differing timespans for repeat EPD.

Aiming for February and March is the best time for pollen/grass desensitisation and before autumn dampness for Candida, though everything is dealt with in each injection whenever it is given. A wet, warm, humid summer can be as miserable as a heavy pollen count. In warm weather, mercury either still in teeth fillings or afterwards as bonded tissue mercury is still susceptible to temperature variations. That's why mercury is used in thermometers because it expands and rises in heat, so it acts similarly in humans during hot weather causing increased lethargy and sinus reactions. Sinusitis has long been a mercury symptom noted amongst early researchers.

TREATMENT

For ten days before EPD treatment, a full course of appropriate anti-fungal preparation like Sporanox, must be taken. De-Nol, which is used in gastric ulcer treatment, is also taken to reduce the ability of Candida to adhere to mucosal linings of the intestinal tract.

Once Candida levels have been reduced, there is a 24-36 hour semi-fast before the injection which reduces all allergenic responses in addition to Candida. (There are only permitted foods and mineral water at this time, and for another 24-36 hours after the injection). These two or three days (including being asleep overnight) are not particularly pleasant because of withdrawal symptoms, like craving, headache, faintness and weakness, but they do vary from person to person and in any case are worth every discomfort once the de-sensitisation takes effect. Eating lamb, carrots, potato, cabbage and banana is not a culinary treat but keeping occupied between meals helps a lot to take one's mind off it and help time to pass. Following the injection are three weeks of carefully designed and very specific vitamin/mineral supplements. Protection appears from 2-4 weeks later and life lifts once more.

This treatment may work totally for some after only two years of treatments, never needing an injection ever again; other severe cases, like me, take much longer to reach the stage of seldom, if ever, needing one again.

Probiotic preparations

From chapter 2, we know that there are friendly bacteria in the intestines, as well as those causing infections. Since the two groups exert a natural control over each other because living space and species survival are the natural law of an eco-system, it would seem sensible to aim at enhancing the friendly group. This reduces risks of bacterial infection, yet controls yeast/Candida levels. Some sort of bacteria has to control the yeast, and it might as well be the friendly sort. These produce acetic and lactic acids which, in turn, promote a more acid environment unfriendly to Candida. For these two reasons, controlling and acidising, lactobacilli and bifidobacteria serve Candida sufferers well. But be warned! Over-use of probiotics will upset the balance! It's a more harmonious balance we need, not an elimination of toxinous bacteria and yeast! Furthermore, research shows that lactobacillus acidophilus actually forms a natural antibiotic during its competitiveness with other bacteria. This production is not only enhanced by an acid environment of pH 5.5, but also when it is taken into the body as a treatment within a yoghurt or milk foodstuff.

Lactobacilli and bifidobacteria produce a substance called 'biotin'. This helps to prevent Candida Albicans from forming hyphae (filaments), which burrow into epithelial cell walls for additional nutrition. In so doing, hyphae scar and damage the walls of the intestines. By creating higher levels of biotin or preserving those which occur naturally, we allow it to protect cell walls and prevent absorption disturbance within villi and capillaries in the small intestines. So how do you know whether to take acidophilus and bifidobacteria? I believe this should be regarded as a treatment, which is why it is discussed in this section. When Candida upsurges and you become aware of it anywhere, either systemically or at local sites, treatment has to start. These friendly bacteria are readily available by mail-order or pharmacies and health-food shops.

If you suffer constantly despite the vital, daily self-help we shall be looking at shortly, then it may be due to past gut damage, antibiotics, amalgams, serious illness, constant tiredness, etc., and all these may necessitate lifestyle changes. In a stressful situation (e.g. job, illness, accident, relationship), adrenaline, which helps to dilate blood vessels and helps the heart and lungs to cope, creates alkalinity (another reason why asthmatics and bronchitis sufferers get so much Candida). Probiotic therapy would counter the effects of this by promoting an acid balance from lactic and acetic acid production.

TREATMENT ADMINISTRATION

First decide whether this is to be for a particular upsurge or something longer term. If it is required to deal with an upsurge, then, in conjunction with self-help, i.e. removing the reason(s) for the upsurge, you may want to try one of the following:

- As soon as you get up, take three soup spoonfuls of a yoghurt with 'live' bifidus (combination of acidophilus, biotin and bifidobacteria). If you take too much, you will start to fart more than usual about three or four days later! (This points to gut disturbance from excessive yoghurt.) Before lunch and before dinner, take three soup spoons again. Try this for seven to ten days, then reduce the dose to one spoonful before every meal, then a holding dose for a week of two spoonfuls before breakfast.
- If you want stronger assistance, then mix a teaspoonful of the powdered form of acidophilus and bifidobacteria (bifidus) in a small glass (just larger than an egg cup) of lukewarm milk and drink it twenty minutes before breakfast.
- If you want a low-dose, preventive therapy, then take one or two soup spoons of plain yoghurt at breakfast.
- If you need a higher-strength holding therapy because of illness, stress, genetics, allergies, antibiotics, contraceptives, steroids and such, then take the morning, strong-assistance dosage regularly. Don't just take it out of habit. You must have good reason for needing to strive against background difficulties so that 'balance' can stand a better chance.

I am against taking any medicines unless the need is absolute. Taking medications is no proper substitute for being sensible in primary, daily healthcare. I always feel that the Japanese and Chinese habit of wearing medical-style masks to contain their own cold germs and to deprive the virus of the cold air in which it thrives is such a great idea that we all ought to do it. There are many simple things like that which involve no expense at all and which promote good health and prevent annoyance illnesses.

This probiotic approach is systemic. It treats at source - the small intestine - and, when carried within milk or yoghurt, can better withstand the acidity of the stomach before doing its work in the small intestines. It should also help Candida in the mouth and throat if held a little in the mouth prior to swallowing slowly.

We are very fortunate in having the benefit of modern research into probiotic therapy. Its inclusion as a therapy for Candida and yeasts has eased a lot of frustration between doctors and patients, enabled patients to control and treat themselves, and shown a different option for treatment, most probably the best one.

Other treatments

These have been covered to some extent elsewhere but there are other helpful products easily available from the mail-order or pharmacy.

Allicin
This is a compound active against many micro-organisms, including the Candida species. It is available in a synthetic form, but otherwise is derived from garlic. Those, like me, who regard garlic as smelly, anti-social and a purgative, may like to look for any kind of tablet containing more allicin than garlic. If you are a garlic household anyway, this won't matter (you may not suffer from Candida either!).

Aloe Vera
This is an ancient anti-Candida therapy from the desert plant of that name. Desert tribes, contending with heat (though usually dry heat) would have eaten much yoghurt from their animals' milk and had access to Aloe Vera should the need arise. We can learn much from the traditional ways of living healthily in hot climates, and I shall be discussing this shortly.

Biotin
Take this as 500mg tablets or capsules with food. Follow the instructions carefully.

Caprylic Acid
This comes from coconuts and kills yeasts in the intestines. Take three capsules at each meal.

Echinacea
Taken as tablet or tincture, this is a strongly anti-fungal herb.

Germanium

This is very strong, so the dosage must only be between 1 mg and 300mg daily.

Olive Oil

Take one teaspoon a day for the oleic acid, which helps in keeping Candida spores from forming hyphae and burrowing into epithelium.

PRACTICAL TREATMENT

Still dealing with a recognisable upsurge as opposed to daily prevention, there are practical steps to take. We will look at the reasons for these in detail shortly, but for now we need to recap the certain basics Candida requires for survival and growth:

- warmth;
- moisture;
- nutrition (sugar/glucose/alcohol);
- an ill or tired host body.

You also need to look at these circumstances:

- Has your body temperature been elevated, e.g. weather, climate, clothing, bedding, exercising?
- Have you worn sweaty clothing, begun keep-fit classes, gone swimming and much more?
- Have you started snacking, drinking alcohol, found a new cake shop, drunk lots of canned drinks, finished a bar of chocolate daily, etc.?
- Have you taken antibiotics or steroids, had an anaesthetic, become ill, overdone it at work, been partying at the weekend, become worried?
- Which of these basic areas, or any others mentioned elsewhere in the book, have been neglected, forgotten or even started, e.g. a new partner who is sexually transmitting Candida to you, chemotherapy, diabetes, asthma treatments, hay fever sprays, etc.?

If the reason or several reasons for this Candidal upsurge are immediately apparent from a good thinking session, then they must be dealt with straight away. Correct things quickly in the most appropriate way, e.g. drop the boyfriend or use a condom and pressure his drinking habits; throw the rest of the Christmas chocolates away; change the sweat-provoking bedding; stop buying the coca cola or lemonade; go to bed and rest; or whatever else needs to be done.

Genital Candidal upsurge

Once higher levels of Candida are being excreted, they travel forwards along the female perineum towards the vulval area. Entrance then is easy into the urethra, bladder and vagina, so hygiene is important, not just for controlling vaginal thrush, but for preventing urethritis and a secondary route into the bloodstream should there be any skin fissures there.

During a Candida upsurge, genital/perineal/anal hygiene is vital: washing is recommended twice a day, possibly three if the weather is hot and sticky, but not baths! They are hot and wet! Showering is all right, provided that the very last thing you do is face the water flow and, with one foot raised, allow the water to run from front to back cleanly, so that nothing running forward during the course of the shower is allowed to remain on the vulva. Men must retract the foreskin and really clean off the smegma first with soap, and then rinse this off thoroughly. All readers and followers of my work with cystitis will know about the bottle-washing process. This, of course, is the best genital hygiene, and it is equally good for washing off Candida or bacteria. It is described in the next chapter.

Rest is very important. The immune system may be down with another health problem or just tiredness. It doesn't need you to give it any further trouble or abuse - help it! Don't hinder it! And by rest, I mean stretched out on the sofa or in bed with the radio or a book not a sexual partner!

Use a chosen cream or pessary, perhaps one that has been helpful in a previous upsurge. It must be carefully inserted at night, following this procedure:

- Wash your hands thoroughly, then bottle-wash the pelvic area.
- Only after a full bottle wash, (see page 147), should the vagina then be rinsed out with cool water from a second bottle otherwise faecal bacteria get pushed in.
- Once the area has finally been dried with an absorbent wash-cloth (discard it for boiling along with the day's underwear), DO NOT use toilet tissue as it leaves contaminated bits behind. Go to bed and stay there!
- Lying flat and relaxed, reach up to the cervix with the tip of the pessary itself or with the applicator, if cream is used.
- Afterwards, if you feel you should wash hands again, then do so quickly, returning to bed. Otherwise put the applicator on a tissue by the bed for cleaning in the morning. If the cream or pessary is inserted in any other position, the cervix will not be treated and Candida remains on it to travel to the vaginal epithelium when the chance comes.
- Finish the treatment by using a systemic drug or Nystatin for gut Candida control, or choose any of the other treatments already mentioned. Never ignore the lifestyle factors, or the basic reasons will remain and another vaginal or penile upsurge will happen as soon

as the careful, expensive medication therapy stops.

- Wear a pad at night to catch vaginal contents, but in the day when at home, go without underwear to help air access for drying the perineum.

If you think sexual activity caused Candida transference, then condoms should be used once treatment has finished and sex has begun again. Male hygiene and treatment are just as important in clearing any genital upsurge.

If vaginal thrush is a cyclical problem before a period, stop it by inserting a lactic acid pessary each night in the preceding week of the period. It may also be helpful during the period and for two or three days after, since blood is alkaline and so is the vagina at this time. The arrival of progestogen to help the uterus to shed its lining is the reason for an alkaline vagina. This occurs naturally or when the contraceptive pill controls the four-week cycles.

Genital Candidal upsurge may also be caused by hormone imbalance, contraceptive choice or the Pill. When or if it upsurges, think back to any change of contraceptive, such as the coil string or the diaphragm (cap) which might harbour thrush. The coil string situation will be helped by good perineal hygiene, lactic acid pessaries or cider vinegar. The diaphragm should be cleaned thoroughly as directed, dried properly and stored correctly in a clean box. Did thrush only begin upon commencing an oral contraceptive? This can cause increased body fluid retention with impaired sugar metabolism and excess sugar. Treat it by systemic self-help for a while, but if thrush fails to improve, the Pill brand may need changing.

Some women prefer a cider vinegar application both before a period or if there is a thrush upsurge at any other time. It can be soaked into a tampon or added to the vaginal bottle wash.

If Candida is causing urethritis in either sex, hygiene is vital once urine tests or uncomfortable urethral swabs have proved positive. Systemic treatment will be prescribed, or you can use any of the other plans mentioned already. Cream for the penis and all around and underneath the foreskin will have to be applied with as much dedication as for the vagina. Candida of the penis is caused by identical reasons to vulval candida, but can also be found in alcohol drinkers, sweaty athletes or dancers, victims of MDS, swimmers or joggers.

Thrush upsurge in the mouth and throat

Treatment for these sites takes second place to knowing the cause, which may be:

- general ill health;

- oral/genital Candidal transference during intercourse;
- steroid inhalers for rhinitis or asthma;
- sweets /chocolates/canned drinks/alcohol;
- yeast extract on bread or toast;
- dirty or ill-fitting dentures; dental treatment generally;
- an old toothbrush;
- breast milk.

The first step in any treatment must obviously be to withdraw the cause. Easy causes, such as an old toothbrush, yeast extract, oral/ genital sex, sweets, etc. are instantly removable, but there are still the symptoms to treat. With illness of any kind or steroid inhalants, the underlying factors will dictate the cessation or continuation of Candida. Again, comfort levels need elevating, and symptoms of Candida need to be relieved. Babies frequently get thrush in the mouth because the mother has it perhaps from pasta, floury foods, sugary drinks etc,and is passing it on in her milk. If the mother is treated, the baby will improve.

The sucking of an anti-fungal lozenge, as directed by the prescribing doctor, will help a lot. Lemon juice on a cloth as an acid may be worth wiping round affected spots or diluted for gargling. Plain yoghurt (as previously mentioned) can be held a spoonful at a time in the mouth before a slow swallow down the throat. Any of the appropriate probiotic treatments or herbal/nutritional preparations can be tried. However, none will be completely effective if underlying causes are not withdrawn. Don't binge on yoghurt as it can upset gut bacterial balance.

Candidosis of the skin

Treatment for this should be topical (localised) using anti-fungal creams from conventional or alternative sources. Finding a cause is once again all-important or else it will recur. Think about whether:

- you live in a warm, damp house
- your house is in a marshy, high-humidity location
- your house or job is in, or near to, woods or forests
- your job is in a moisture-laden atmosphere
- your job involves sweating or working with water
- your job involves wearing sweaty plastic/rayon/nylon overalls/gloves
- your hobby is a water sport of any kind
- your sport involves getting hot and sweaty

- your recreational jogging takes you into mouldy woods or damp commons
- you deal with animals
- you wear trainers a lot

Systemic treatments and strict attention to self-help may turn the yeast upsurge around so that no further upsurges occur afterwards. If recurrence is a misery, check and remove the lifestyle cause(s).

Only time and situation-recall can begin to tell you which, if any, of these treatment plans you need. It is obvious that Candida can be so mild in some people as to be unnoticeable; equally obvious are those seriously ill or dying patients who are being taken over by rampant Candida. In between the two are countless individual levels of suffering. This whole book and this chapter in particular offer options. There *are* treatment options, and only you, the doctor or patient, can decide upon an individually usefully type.

10 Daily living

We only have one body each and it is our responsibility. It is sickening to have to deal constantly with health problems, and this is made far worse by meeting people who always seem to be in the peak of health and seldom ill. It simply doesn't seem fair. There they are, partying, drinking, eating whatever they like, needing little sleep, full of energy for a demanding job after a night on the tiles. But it's no use wishing it otherwise. However it may seem, everyone has some kind of health trouble somewhere, some weakness, some kind of impediment. You may not know about it and you may never be told. If Candida is your misery, get on with it, be practical and accept susceptibility to upsurges.

Caring for this sensitivity is not time-consuming, painful or costly if you are sensible. There are drugs and therapies available if you let yourself down, so there is no need to panic in bad times, though if a bad time comes, it does take time, patience and money to beat it. Candida retreats slowly and is far best avoided in the first place.

The daily prevention of Candida is absolutely no different to preventing lots of health problems. We all take things like visits to the dentist and optician, washing, grooming, exercising in our stride, as part of our daily rituals, yet these all contribute to preventing health problems. Don't grumble about Candida - it may seem an all-consuming problem, and it certainly can be, but is that because you have, as yet, no good way of keeping it under control? Have you only done restrictive, miserable, impractical diets? Have you spent a fortune on supplements and realised this is not only costly but depressing to contemplate for ever?

The answer is probably yes. Over the years, many such people have trodden a last-ditch path to my counselling door and not one of them has looked at the reasons WHY. Unless there is full, frank and untimed (up to three hours) disclosure of the entire lifestyle, there can be no sure path to prevention and release from future upsurges of Candida.

My personal and professional knowledge of Candida counts a great deal in helping other sufferers. I spoke personally in chapter 1 of my early frustrations as a Candida sufferer. There has had to be a practical, reasonable way of dealing with it, so that it is not only controlled by me, but kept firmly at a level where it doesn't worry or control me. I know my own trigger factors and their levels.

Caring for your body

So, viruses and illnesses apart, we must now look at the small but vital acts of body care that go such a long way to reducing the chances of Candidal upsurge. They are vital at all levels of upsurge, whether mild, medium or severe. Each level can be reduced by several steps to prevent any upsurges at all, turning a moderate upsurge into something milder or reducing something nasty into something less traumatic. We must once again remember the basic requirements for Candida Albicans to upsurge, colonise and gain control. It needs:

* warmth;
* moisture;
* sugar, glucose or alcohol to feed on;
* tired, stressed or sick host body;
* bacteria-to-yeast imbalance.

Whilst fully acknowledging that the mucosal areas of the body are regulated somewhat beyond our control, it must be equally obvious that what we wear or eat and the jobs or hobbies we pursue must influence our body as outside factors. These we are definitely able to control or change ourselves. Indeed, in years of Candida counselling, I know how exceptionally important and beneficial these ideas and practicalities are for every single Candida sufferer.

> Rachel had a new boyfriend. He was a ball player for the town team and after each game the bar became a focal point for their early-relationship entertainment. Disliking beer, she drank copious juices and sodas instead! After four weeks of this new social drinking, she began to feel hot, sore and itchy between the legs. Her mouth became roughened and dry, and her sinuses stuffy. From a session with me, this new social order was deemed culpable. Rachel is back to water or orange squash (not juice) and, together with a look at her alcohol intake after work, she has seen the light! Sugar and alcohol levels were reduced and her symptoms disappeared.

Other than plain yoghurt (three spoonfuls three times a day), she needed no treatment as such. The removal of the cause was the answer. Whilst in counselling, I took her over other basic rules for prevention of vaginal thrush.

DIET

- Reduce or remove all sugars, chocolates, yeast extract, mushrooms, cheese, cakes, biscuits, gateaux, fruit (although bananas are OK), canned or bottled drinks (except still mineral water), alcohol or non-alcohol drinks, vinegars, French dressing (made with vinegar) and yeasty foods.
- Cut out all caffeine to reduce natural steroid/hormone production.
- Check out your chosen form of contraception.

PASTIMES

Any sport, hobby or pastime can, in a sensitive person, add a possibility of Candida upsurge.

Swimming

This involves Lycra swimwear which, once used, should be changed and rinsed well to expel as much pool antiseptic and chlorine as possible. The pool water itself has had its levels of chlorine and antiseptics heavily raised, especially in inner cities. Much vaginal yeast infection occurs because pool water is now a heavy antibiotic/antiseptic mixture removing bacteria from perineal and vaginal skin Once the natural bacterial levels are regularly lowered, Candida surges.

Keep fit/aerobics

Another very common cause of vaginal thrush, lycra outfits are again one of the reasons. No air at all is allowed onto the perineum. A double blow is dealt by elevated body temperatures during the workout. Thrush loves it! No air and plenty of heat and sweat! Ideally you should wear cotton, exercise moderately and then do a cool-water bottle wash afterwards to cool down the vulva and perineum. All sports can elevate body temperature. Either change to a less exacting sport, give up Lycra clothing, cool off with a cool-water bottle wash and leave off pants or give it up totally if you can pinpoint it as the cause of constant vaginal thrush from reading this book.

BUSINESS

Much of today's increased incidence of vaginal thrush can be attributed to modern business technology. Computers, typewriters, phone lines, meetings and more all keep women sitting down for lengthy blocks of time. Work entailing being seated all the time, except for lunch, doesn't help vaginal health. Weight pivots upon the vulval area from pressure of the seat upwards and from downward pressure of the upper body. From below and above, this pressure traps blood in the sensitive vulval network. On standing, this trapped heat causes swelling and discomfort. There can clearly be no air access at all for the hours during which the perineum is subjected to such treatment. If underwear is nylon and hygiene poor, bacteria and yeasts will reproduce nicely in the warmth and moisture.

Another business hazard for women is going to the bar for a 'quick one' at lunch or after work. Remember, alcohol is a major cause of Candida.

Tight skirts and false modesty force the wearer to keep her legs together when walking and when sitting elegantly with legs crossed. Air is again denied to the perineum. Trousers, too, prevent sufficient air reaching the vulval area.

> Beverley was the lead singer in a great all-girls group. She danced, too, at gigs up and down the country, three or four times a week. She wore a lot of black, leather outfits and body stockings. At the interval and after the show, she would cool down with pints of iced cola. Levels of vaginal and intestinal Candida were consequently high, life such a misery that her boyfriend was threatening to go, and she was barely able to get through each gig from the pain, soreness and irritation.
>
> After three hours of counseling, she went away with a complete revision of hygiene, show clothing, liquid intake and ideas to cool down. Improvements began straight away, and with little medication, except oral nystatin and vaginal pessaries for the first ten days, she gained control over the situation. Prevention took over from the medications and enabled her to keep the boyfriend, do the gigs and prevent future Candidal upsurge.
>
> Linda's enjoyment two or three times a week was swimming. She either swam with friends near her home in the country or she used a larger, busier pool downtown. Vaginal thrush plagued her. She decided that since she couldn't get to grips with it, she would come for counseling. From her diaries, it was possible to see that when she swam in the clear pool in Harrow, there was no resulting upsurge, but when she was up in London using the milky, heavily chlorinated pool in Holborn, there would be an upsurge a week later.
>
> From deciding only to swim at Harrow and clean out the vagina carefully afterwards, vaginal thrush was defeated yet again by precise, personalised prevention.

CLOTHING

This must not prevent air access to the perineum. The perineum (between the legs) is a warm, moist area anyway, so we don't want to make it more so by trapping sweat or creating extra. This means:

- no jeans;
- loose 'baggies' occasionally;
- no nylon underwear (or nylon underneath a cotton gusset!);
- no tights;
- no panty-girdles, body stockings or corsets;
- no panty liners;
- no tampons (except in the cider vinegar therapy);
- no Lycra leotards;
- no riding breeches;
- no tight office skirts.

At home, especially in hot weather, wear a loose dress or skirt without underwear. In cold weather, wear long vests, longer skirts or culottes made from warm, natural material like wool, warm stockings with a suspender belt, waist slips, heavy cotton briefs. In other words, keep as warm as you like with natural, warm clothing, but cover the immediate perineal area with just one layer of breathing cotton. Even in the coldest weather, so long as other warm clothing is worn, the occasional hour at home without underwear can be very helpful.

Hygiene

Sexually active women need to keep pubic hair cut every five or six weeks to about an inch and a half in length. All hair follicles secrete oil and moisture, as well as trapping and receiving yeasts. Once trapped, the nutrients in the sweat serve as food, and Candida can colonise.

PERINEAL CLEANING

In many areas of the world, water, especially clean water, is scarce. Small amounts for washing are a luxury and have to be used with maximum efficiency. Religious reasons frequently account for water usage, for instance, Muslims must wash genitalia and hands before praying. This is largely symbolic these days, but the idea was not only to be clean when prostrate in Allah's presence, but also to get rid of dirt at opportune times in the working day. Before water came on tap in these places, milk from the goats or sheep was used for washing, or even sterile sand for cleaning the hands and anus.

In short, water scarcity brought a reverence for liquids which never materialised in areas blessed with plenteous water. As a result of piped water into homes this century, we have all become used to splashing it about and taking it for granted. Re-cycling in cities is the only way to provide a growing population's habit of daily baths, twice-daily showers or whatever. Yet there are enormous gaps in our knowledge about how to use this vital liquid efficiently.

The area between our legs is hardly enormous. A bath or a shower is not essential to cleaning such a small area (we would hardly want to use garden shears to cut our toe nails!). Yet the female perineum is undoubtedly the second highest at-risk area for transmittance of infection after the mouth. Micro-organisms from our own faecal expulsion abound here. Even when we pass wind, millions more are propelled out of the anus and deposited on underwear, nightwear, sanitary towels, etc. to then swim around in micro-droplets of moisture.

For sufferers of Candida (and/or cystitis), hygiene is of very great importance in cleaning this muck off regularly. However, don't rush off to buy a bidet, since every single kind, from those with gold-leaf jets to plastic portable car bidets, are unspeakably dangerous! They should really be banned or carry government health warnings!

Reasons for not using bidets

- Germs and spores run forwards with gravity.
- Germs and spores run everywhere.
- Putting in a plug and sitting in the organisms will contaminate you.
- Temperature levels are impossible to control.
- Central sprays blast bacteria everywhere.
- It is seldom understood that facing the taps is the correct way to sit.
- Despite facing the taps, water cannot run upwards and round a curve to reach the anus behind.
- Even if it does, it runs with gravity back towards the vagina and urethra.

Thankfully bidets are considered a luxury, and few homes have one. Do not use a Bidet! Anywhere!

BOTTLE-WASH

This is primarily done after a bowel movement, which is when the greatest amounts of Candida and bacteria emerge onto the perineum. The timing of passing a stool therefore becomes important. Those who regularly perform after breakfast in their own home are lucky. Those with sporadic bowel movements, often at work, need to keep a toiletry bag at work containing the simple items needed. If you get 'caught short' whilst shopping, either bottle-wash as soon as you reach personal surroundings or, if some time has yet to elapse before this is possible, use a green paper towel or kitchen roll to wet-wipe reasonably well. Bottle-wash properly as soon as you get home. Manufactured wet-wipes or medicated wipes contain chemicals and antiseptics which may affect a tender perineum. They must not be used.

Tissues or soft toilet paper must not be used for drying off after a bottle-wash. They disintegrate immediately in any moisture, spreading contamination as you walk and chafing. To use them is to run a great risk of increasing Candida colonies or faecal bacterial infections. In a 'shopping' emergency, use with great care and wash properly when you get home.

How to bottle-wash correctly

Apart from a toilet and a hand basin, you only need:

- a bar of ordinary soap (sensitive-skinned people should use a plain, uncoloured, unperfumed, non-antiseptic brand);
- one or two bottles 500mls, not less, not more. It must be a tonic or soda bottle, not a milk bottle, which needs re-sterilizing, or anything larger or smaller;
- a wash- cloth for drying

Some women think they can improve upon these simple yet specific items. Change them at your peril! The amount of water, the bottle size and type, the wash-cloth are all vital and specific. Don't use mugs, jugs, watering cans, shower gels, toilet paper or any variations.

The method

1 Pass a stool and use toilet paper until this becomes clean.
2 Flush the toilet, stand up but don't pull your pants up..
3 Turn on both hot and cold taps (**don't** put the basin plug in), wash your hands and scrub under your nails briefly.
4 Re-soap one hand very well. Still standing up, thoroughly soap the back passage with this soapy hand. *Don't* use the bar of soap for this purpose, *don't* soap further forward, and *don't* use wipes, cloths or cotton wool.
5 Rinse that hand under the hot, running tap.
6 Now fill one or two 500m1 bottles with warm water, (warmer than lukewarm). Mix the hot and cold until the temperature in the bottle is right. Turn the taps off now.

7   Return to the toilet and sit down *centrally*.

8   Position yourself, buttocks apart. Flop your backbone down and the anus will follow, being then the lowest part of the perineum so that water falls off the anal opening and cannot run uphill to the genitals. This is called a pelvic tilt.

9   *From the front*, using the left hand, pour the warm bottle of water between your legs. You *must* use your other hand to clean the genitals and then reach downwards to clean away *completely* all traces of the soap which now contains all the bacteria. Use the second bottle if all the soap hasn't gone.

10 Stand up and pat the perineum dry with the wash-cloth. Keep this apart on its own hook (although there aren't any germs on it. They are down the toilet). Don't use paper or cotton wool for drying.

Remember, faecal material is greasy. It will only come off with warm water and soap!

Common mistakes in Bottle-Washing

- Not enough soap on the hand.
- Bottles too big or too small, milk bottles that should have been sterilised, jugs that pour badly. Use **only** 500ml bottles (e.g. Schweppes); they have been carefully chosen and researched.
- Not sitting on the toilet with the anus as the lowest point.
- Leaning back against the toilet cistern. You just can't reach the backpassage from this position, and it clenches the buttocks, preventing water from a clear, backward flow.
- Using cotton wool or a cloth to soap the anus. Don't! You contaminate yourself, block up the toilet, miss the skin folds and haemorrhoids. Only soap with your hands, so that all nooks and crannies get soapy.
- Using a bidet. A bidet is dangerous, it spreads bacteria around. Never use one!
- Putting the basin plug in and rinsing your hands in a solution of faecal bacteria.
- Not doing it every time you open your bowels and thinking that missing it once will be all right!
- Standing in the bath with one leg on the edge and trying to shower the perineum.

This is the basic bottle-washing technique to which I have referred in other parts of this book, such as before inserting an anti-fungal cream or pessary at night. If the perineum is not cleared of Candida beforehand, then the cream, applicator or pessary will certainly push additional Candida and bacteria into the vagina. Bottle Washing must be done without fail before any kind of sexual intercourse, before inserting creams or pessaries, after a bowel movement.

Cool-water bottle-washing procedure (after a full one !)

1 Wash your hands and fill the 500 ml bottle with coolish water, not hot.
2 Sit on the toilet and pass urine.
3 Now do the pelvic tilt (backbone downwards).
4 From the front, slowly pour the tepid water down the perineum and clean it.
5 Insert the largest finger of your other hand into the vagina and reach to the cervix, hooking out secretions as the water is trickling (you may need to do this five or six times) so that this coolness cleans and calms the vagina. Use a second bottle, if needed.
6 Stand up and pat dry with the wash-cloth kept for perineal drying.
7 Rest for at least ten minutes with your feet up and no underwear! Best of all, go to bed for a good night's sleep. Drink a glass of water.
8 If you've had a heavy sex session, you might benefit from the above cool-water bottle. Wash again in the morning.
9 Insert cream or pessary into the cervix.

Once all sexual activity has ceased, nothing more can actually cause soreness, bruising or irritation unless you take a hot bath, pull on a pair of jeans, go riding or even do a three-mile walk. The simple, but incredibly effective, cool-water bottle-wash stops all trouble.

Bottle-washing is applicable to all women of any age, though small girls should only require a daily bath (not too hot, and no bubble bath!). Bottle-washing is only a modernised version of ancient perineal washing routines and will control Candida movement from anus to vulva. Hot or long baths will increase irritation inflammation and Candida colonies. If the above advice is followed, underwear is changed daily, bottle washing is regular; the vagina is cleaned out with a second bottle of cooler water and discharge hooked out with the longest finger of the other hand not holding the bottle; pubic hair is kept to an inch and a half long; air is accessed to the perineum then anti-fungal control of vaginal thrush by self-help is extremely effective.

The boiling and ironing of underwear becomes needless when greater attention is paid to specific hygiene.

Prevention of bladder Candida

It must be obvious, since the vagina and urethra lie upon each other and share the joint exit point of the vulva, that anything affecting the vagina can also affect the urethra. Ascending micro-organisms like Candida love the warmth and moisture.

They can sometimes survive the mildly acidic urethral epithelium and normal mild acidity of the regularly flushed bladder.

Every rule for perineal hygiene applies equally in substance and response to the urethra and bladder as it does to the vagina. Likewise diet and clothing count every bit as much, if not more. The bladder receives waste products in liquid urine. Sugar excess, particularly in diabetics, can cause redness and soreness, which basically shows up as a Candidal presence. If attention is paid to removal of sugar from the diet and to sensible cool-water bottle washing, which will remove excessive surface sugar levels, then progress can be made.

Prevention of intestinal and systemic Candida

The incidence of intestinal and systemic Candidosis can usually be related to the sufferer's lifestyle somewhere. This means that prevention is possible. Every chapter in the book except this one deals with *medical* causes followed by treatment.

This chapter deals with *self-inflicted* causes followed by preventive removal of those causes. Many have already been addressed because, by and large, local sites of Candida upsurge are only external manifestations of what is going on in the intestines. There are varying levels of severity in systemic Candidosis. Doctors easily find chronic Candidosis in obviously sick or dying patients but they have trouble acknowledging or proving its presence on a less severe level in other patients.

There appear to be hundreds of thousands of people unable to gain credence or acceptance as systemic Candida victims because the obvious is apparently not medically obvious. Disbelief reigns in every surgery in the land. Until science catches up with the sufferers, I believe it is an affront to the sufferer not to recognise their own account and personal body knowledge by refusing and withholding systemic treatment.

That being clearly stated, I want to move on to personal prevention. This allows for personal knowledge and control to a very great extent over intestinal or systemic Candida. To disregard this and to rely only on systemic or localised treatment is an abuse of the drugs and of medical health care. Only when patients and doctors trust each other and value the specific help with which each side supports the other can any of us hope to move away from a total treatment and prescription approach. The doctor/practitioner has every right to expect patient participation in prevention, and if this is understood, then support, when necessary with appropriate drugs, can be added.

General health

When illness strikes more often because we all live in closer proximity to each other, travel more and eat out more often, we are in greater contact with viruses. Life can become miserable sometimes. It is not a cause for depression. It is a time to re-state the rules, show patience with the sick body, care for it, rest it, comfort and treat it. This body is your friend, and you must fight for it and support it. Candidal upsurge is a secondary reaction to some part of your daily life that is not in tune with what your healthy body requires.

TIREDNESS

Don't ignore it! Tiredness is a warning that the body requires rest. Candida-prone people cannot afford to be tired or to feel tired for very long. If there has been, or might be, a period of intense activity, prolonged stress, prolonged illness or even winter blues, you must make a management plan and a recovery plan.

Management Plan

- Early bed-times with 'aided' sleep.
- Don't have cocoa or chocolate drinks before going to bed.
- Don't drink alcohol, e.g. brandy or whisky, before bed; it will backfire on you the next day with all the known side-effects.
- Ease any stress by 'dropping' it for an hour or so. See a movie or join an interesting class for writing or languages or birdwatching, anything!
- Talk to a close friend, making sure to listen to their problems, too.
- Take a general mineral and/or vitamin supplement for a month.
- Maybe get an iron blood count taken.
- Take a pleasant walk, either a short, energetic one or a lengthier, social one with a friend.
- Sit in the garden or a park with a book or newspaper.
- If you are sad and grieving, restrict the crying to several shorter periods. One long, uninterrupted one will increase tiredness and mineral/vitamin depletion from heavy fluid loss.
- Change the job, re-work better hours, stop the night shift, stop the affair.
- If sadness is likely to last, try to make one plan a day to keep sad thoughts from penetrating. The immune system needs this break badly.
- Something physical is usually helpful.
- If sleep patterns are badly thrown, then get up, eat a slice of toast and have a herbal drink, read five pages of a book and try again with the lights out.
- If, as with ME or any other serious illness, sleep patterns cease to exist and are all over the

place, then sleeping pills or herbal remedies on alternate nights or to break a recent run of bad nights may be needed. Take sparingly, since the mind can learn to rely on them. Get the mercury amalgams out safely as they can cause insomnia.

- Long, soaky baths cause mineral and vitamin loss from opened pores. They are also very hot and wet and Candida likes this!
- Do everything you can to remedy the illness as quickly as possible and get well so that tiredness is minimalised.

Recovery Plan

- Make sure that particular set of circumstances is unlikely to recur.
- Take a break.
- Stay with a quiet-living friend, not a partying kind, if it is illness from which you need to recover.
- If it is recovery from grieving or sadness, then a partying friend might be just the ticket!
- Long, seaside walks are great for helping with sleep, thoughts, energy levels or weight gain. Autumn, winter or spring are exceptionally good times. Summer is too hot and wearing.
- Stare at a fire, light a couple of candles each night.
- See a show one night a week.
- Join a choir and use your lungs.
- Enjoy a fancied treat (not a bar of chocolate).

Much of this is practical, much of it uplifting. A bright outfit can also do wonders for morale. Wear yellows or reds to bolster flagging energy. If black or grey are normal colours for you, then go and buy some bright tops and sweaters. Put out a bowl of oranges or red apples - anything that brings sunshine into your surroundings. At a day-course in colour I once attended, the lecturer, after peering at each participant in turn, gave separate colour needs for each of us. I was told to buy tangerines and look at them in front of me. I didn't just look, I held one in each hand for the rest of the day, and it felt wonderful, my eyes and hands just drank the colour in. Try it if you are feeling drained. If it's peace and tranquillity you need, then blues and greens, like staring at a field or a sky, wearing a blue or green scarf or top can achieve this.

If you have to go into hospital, take a variety of colours to wear or touch or look at. My red hot-water bottle is my staple comfort! Red flowers in a vase or orange fruit in a bowl are tremendous elevators of courage, assurance, decisiveness and energy. Eat colourful food. Design and plan meals with colour schemes, such as pink.

- avocado with pink mayonnaise sauce followed by
- lamb with red-oak lettuce salad, a sherry glass of rose wine and
- strawberry creme pots with pink wafer biscuits

How about an orange theme-

- carrot soup followed by
- chicken livers in orange sauce with sliced oranges and orange capsicum salad
- then brandy baskets filled with macaroon and peaches.

Choose recipes appropriate to where your recovery is now. Do a small supper or lunch for friends with a colour theme. Candle and napkin colours can team up spectacularly with a specially arranged menu to match.

When I was included in a research study of people likely or proven to be mercury toxic or allergic from their amalgams, part of the research was aimed at finding out how we coped with such severe health trauma and its resulting depression. I answered that, after two years in bed, I put a date up for ending it all if no solution was forthcoming. I was some nine months into my 'final' year when Bee Propolis in high doses began to put me on my feet. Life appeared again, but all through that dreadful time, I realised that harmless 'treats' were going to save my mind and spirit. I'm sure they did, and many of you will find something here to recognise and value. The Bee Propolis was a temporary help; only full safe amalgam removal ended nearly nine years mainly bedbound.

Tiredness can be physical and mental. Don't allow it to linger, don't accept it, it will pull your immune system down, and Candida, if you are prone, may well upsurge. Enjoy a good laugh, too!

BOWELS

We know well enough by now that excreting waste and micro-organisms is important for controlling Candidal activity. If bowels and peristalsis are sluggish, yeasts and bacteria stay longer, breed faster and obtain maximum nutrition. If they are not allowed to linger, these internal benefits are withdrawn. With the external benefits of the bottle, washing off residual, microscopic, perineal yeast contamination, we hit them again.

Many individual ways of achieving regular bowel movements are on offer. If you have one already, keep going, but if there are difficulties, such as a need for strong purgatives, colonic irrigations, suppositories or just needing a change and alternative, then here are some suggestions:

- Eat oat bran, e.g. a bowl of porridge, every morning.
- Eat two or three dried prunes at breakfast (even add to the oats if experimenting proves valuable).
- Drink a glass of hot or cold water from a flask as soon as you wake.
- Take a hot, pre-breakfast shower.
- Eat muesli with a little, occasional wheat bran added.
- Eat a cooked breakfast followed by a hot-water drink (not coffee or tea).
- Take a good, brisk walk every day.
- Get excited about something! Don't 'put it off'. Find a toilet! Let peristalsis do the work and the stool will be soft, quick and satisfying!
- Take a familiar herbal laxative.
  (Older people may need this on alternate nights, others not so regularly. It's all down to individual experiment and your own 'normality'.)
- Eat an apple or a small orange a day. Candida sufferers are not allowed more fruit than this per day because of high fruit sugar.
- Fibogel or other such gentle products are always best for occasional help.
- Colonic irrigations are expensive and not needed when there is a daily bowel movement.
- Purgatives only add to regulation upheaval.
- Finally, think about it! Get in the mood! Try and get it as a habit, sparked off at a regular time each day, such as after meals.
- Don't put it off for a minute if you are busy, or the moment will be lost!
- Cut out all sugar and caffeine.

If haemorrhoids are either dormant or currently a problem, they will benefit greatly from regular bowel movements that do not pressure them. Older people, pregnant women, even young people are prone to haemorrhoids and, of course, the irregular surfaces of bowel lining, anal skin and swollen blood vessels are great harbours for yeasts and bacteria. Very careful bottle-washing cleans it all off. Candidal upsurge can trigger swollen haemorrhoids because of the itense irritation. Variations on Irritable Bowel Syndrome where diarrhoea alternates with hard 'cherry stones' can and should be managed. The minute a spell of this starts, take any of your prescribed medications, change diet if necessary and pull the wretched bowels back to normal by using any of the recommendations here or your own 'best shots'. Avoid letting trouble settle in. Hit it hard and fast, but sensibly. IBS benefits from safe mercury amalgam removal early on. Otherwise it may lead to serious surgery and a limited life quality. Crohn's Disease is serious and sufferers will be under intense medical care. When it is first diagnosed do get mercury amalgam safely removed, don't wait on until the colostomy becomes necessary.

FARTING

This activity is not simply embarrassing; it also blasts air-borne micro-organisms onto bedding, nightwear, underwear and, of course, the perineum. Since micro-droplets of moisture exit as well, there is immediate perineal travel of organisms.

Farting is also a common symptom of yeast/Candidal infestations. It is likely to be found in some vegetarians, most beer drinkers, sufferers from intestinal parasites such as Giardia, cheese eaters and sugar addicts. Remove or restrict the reason(s) for it, keep bowels regular and bottle-wash the perineum exactly as described. The female should always do a full Bottle Wash before sex and her partner take a full overhead shower. After sex pass urine and do a cool-water bottle-wash to remove heat and inflammation.

Farting causes Candida expulsion onto the perineum and helps it to travel forwards to the vulva. The healthy regularity of peristalsis and bowel movements cannot be stressed too strongly when controlling Candida Albicans.

TOILETS AND LAUNDERING

It is worthwhile pausing here to consider that it is not just our own bodies which need to be kept washed and clean. I've had more than enough women, especially young women, in for counselling on both cystitis and Candida to know that there can be serious discrepancies in standards of bathroom cleanliness.

Cleaning the toilet only once a week is absolutely unacceptable. It must be done daily if more than one person uses it. Single people should aim at once a day, but may be forgiven if cleaning is done on alternate days. For wider use, all bathroom equipment - toilet, basin, bath and shower - must be attended to each day or extra if required. (Throw out the bidet!)

I find that the main problem during the cleaning process itself is that people keep the cleaning cloth scrunched up in a wadge during rinsing. How can cleaning fluid and whatever it has removed off the equipment be truly rinsed if tap water simply cannot reach much of the cloth? Open it out to its fullest extent and let water run through every fibre. Rub it together and hold it again under hot running tap water. When it runs clear without bubbles, it is ready for rinsing equipment.

All sanitary ware surfaces must have cleaning fluid deposits properly removed. If not, then skin reactions may result from using the bath or the toilet. When the cloth has been finally rinsed through, it needs to be allowed to dry as quickly as possible. Bacteria and yeast deposits remaining in the fibres can cling and survive in moisture. Spread the cloth out over some structure that has air access underneath and on top. Mine covers an antique chamber pot; perhaps two hooks for either side of the cloth protruding well away from a wall, might work. One peg means that the cloth hangs closely in folds and cannot dry quickly.

An absorbent, cotton, string cloth is best, not J-cloths, sponges or polyester type cloths, and a regular household surface cleaner is all right. Use a sturdy toilet brush around the bowl before starting on rim and seat with the cloth. Every so often, blitz the bowl with something stronger.

Bathrooms abound with faecal residual bacteria and yeasts; science shows residue to be found up to six feet away from a flushed toilet. Using a strange toilet is not a problem at all if you line the seat with toilet paper before using it. This allows a full, relaxed urinary flow or bowel movement and acts as an impromptu bacterial barrier.

Laundering of underwear for Candida sufferers is no problem whatsoever when that person is doing proper bottle-washing. If the vaginal drip from curdy Candidal discharge is being washed out, after a full bottle-wash, by a cool vaginal bottle-wash, then discharge will be far less likely to emerge onto the vulva. Two such vaginal wash-outs a day not only remove the Candida, but also keep underwear in a better, yeast-free state. Failure to bottle-wash will certainly allow discharge onto underwear. During an upsurge of vaginal, urethral, penile or bladder Candidal upsurge, underwear must be changed each day and need not be laundered separately. It should be dried and aired thoroughly before wearing again.

Underwear should look nice, smell nice and be clean. Every so often, throw it away and buy good cotton replacements, one for each day of the week.

ENVIRONMENT

Jim travelled for his job several times a year. The oil industry, in which he worked, took him to a variety of climates, from very cold and dry to very hot and humid. Every time he travelled to Houston in Texas and every time he travelled to Lagos, Nigeria, he came back with itchy ears. In his sleep, his little finger scratched to relieve the irritation, and after a few days, a watery discharge, smelling distinctively, ran out on to his cheeks and pillow. Ear swabs revealed Candida. After some trips and time had passed by, he and his alert doctor spotted the link with humid climates. As a preventive measure, he took anti-fungal ear drops away with him to humid locations and avoided the onset of a full-blown Candidal infestation. He restricted alcohol and cut out cheese and sugar.

Richard went to a boarding school when he was thirteen. Each weekend the boys had to run for an hour cross-country. This was normally no problem. He liked jogging, but in his first term, the autumn term, the path through the local wood became deep in fallen, rotting Leaves. Dampness and mist rose in the wood' and as the boys crashed through disturbing the fallen Leaves, unseen clouds of fungal spores soared up into the faces of each successive runner. Richard felt his chest tightening, his ears, nose and throat irritating and after fifty yards, he had to stop. On the first time he suffered acutely, and after only two or three more difficult times in the wood, he went to the school doctor. Before the Saturday run, until Christmas, he used an inhaler and also took it with him on the run. Mould spores creating a fungal asthma were then prevented from causing excessive histamine production. Eventually, the doctor sensibly requested an alternative route for Richard away from the wood.

Where you live or work may, because of its dampness and vegetation, be spore-laden with moulds and fungi. This may manifest itself somewhat like summer hay fever, with sneezing and wheezing. Humid weather and rain during a warm spell can bring on sneezing and wheezing, too. It may even cause skin eruptions of Candida or systemic Candida if basic anti-Candida rules are not also taken into account, like no alcohol, no hot baths, no sugars, etc. Any environmental allergy reaction distresses the intricacies of the immune system. Hay fever, gases, fumes, pollens, grasses, dust, industrial emission into the air and more can affect balance of histamines, steroid action, glandular activity, enzyme activity and therefore Candidal levels. Medications to alleviate the symptoms certainly affect body system balances, as we have already discovered. If it comes to it, you may be better to re-locate, or you may prefer desensitisation.

DIET

Too many practitioners in complementary medicines recommend a 'diet only' response to Candida therapy. Rigid, fasting dietary regimes may initially be undertaken by desperate people, but eventually they have to relax them. By this time, patients have become greatly weakened, despite heavy supplementary courses of minerals and vitamins. Our bodies require bulk and substance, as well as nutritional specifics. The basics are contained in three high quality meals a day. Candida sufferers require these more than most people. Something, somewhere in the body is out of balance, either through illness, tiredness, drug therapies, metabolic disturbance, genetic predisposition, mercury poisoning or lifestyle factors and anything else mentioned in this book.

While it is being sorted out, the body requires great assistance to maintain energy. Body activity and immune system support need lots of help. Handfuls of expensive supplements are insufficient. If Candida levels are, in your view, this high, then desensitisation injections and/or safe mercury amalgam removal are more sensible long-term options.

Nevertheless, three good meals a day need a master plan. As far as I am concerned, and therefore anyone here for personal counseling, my prime dietary response to high Candida levels in the intestines is to remove less important foods. These are not 'staple' foods, only extras. A good, high-quality diet does not have to have mushrooms, cream, chocolate, sweets, sugars, canned fruit/drinks, alcohol, yeast extracts, yeasty foods, cakes, gateaux, fizzy drinks, French dressing, vinegars, cheese. Most of these are manufactured taste-bud stimulants, not quality, slow-burning energy givers. We may certainly have developed a taste for them, but that is as a result of advertising, marketing, habit, shopping habit or craving.

> Janet was promoted from her local office to head office in the county town. She worked harder than before and often had to have sandwiches and coffee instead of a decent meal in the little local restaurant, which had been her lunch-hour habit. Now she ate cheese sandwiches or baps, with/without pickles, with/without beetroot, with/without mayonnaise, with/without tomatoes, with/without lettuce. It was cheese all the way, most days. It was washed down with black coffee to 'keep her alert' during the afternoon.
>
> Candida caused a bloated, windy gut and non-stop vaginal soreness. Swabs revealed thrush, and her husband became a sufferer, too. After visiting me, the cheese was stopped the coffee was stopped (since it is an artificial stimulant which depletes energy), sex stopped for a couple of weeks and anti-fungal remedies employed. By reducing the cheese because moulds are introduced to vary the tastes and colours, Janet deprived Candida in the intestines of further yeasty nutrition. Once this was withdrawn, Candida levels declined and all symptoms disappeared.

Cheese and chocolate are, in my counseling experience, two of the top Candida-causing foods. To many people, they appear to be safe, nutritious snacks or meal foods. This may not be true. They can be very damaging to many people. Men frequently order cheese and beer in a pub, as they have done for centuries. Pruritis Ani, that age-old scourge, may well have its origins in beer and cheese - the typical ploughman's lunch. Either refuse all cheese as though it's poisonous (which it may indeed be for you) or have the willpower to restrict it to a mouthful (a small mouthful!) every ten days or so, I manage an occasional cheese topping on a dish or sometimes two biscuits after dinner with a small piece of Brie on each. I will then restrict something else for a couple of days to lower my personal gut Candida levels.

My own gut damage from so many antibiotics, mercury ingested from a mouthful of fillings, lifelong immune system stress and illnesses makes me very vulnerable. Desensitisation by EPD has helped hugely but I still try not to take dietary chances. Chocolate shops fill me with fury. They might just as well say 'Candida Candies'. Chocolate bars, fillings, toppings, Easter eggs, buttons and the like are quick, low-quality, short-term energisers which abuse and upset insulin production, blood sugar levels and cause a huge amount of Candidal misery. They can stop sexual intercourse for long periods until the sufferer understands the cause - no more chocolate! If sweets or chocolates are merely a habit, just don't buy them! Hand them back to the giver or throw them away if they are a present. Never start your children on them. Restrict them and hopefully you won't have a hyperactive little monster on your hands or your conscience! Tooth decay will be prevented, and you will not have to sit in agony whilst your child has to have drilling or extractions.

If you get to grips with less important foods, you will considerably improve daily control of Candida levels.

Other foods

I regard two slices of organic wholewheat bread as acceptable; Soda bread is not since it contains alkaline soda. Look for organics, wheat-free, yeast-free and experiment for yourself. Carbohydrate staples like pasta, rice or potatoes should be varied and rotated daily. They are energizers and are best at breakfast or lunch not evening when the digestive system starts to wind down for the night. High energy foods need to be able to burn off during daytime activites.

Fresh Fruits are best in the morning and help an active digestion and peristalsis. Alternate them. If you are well, try one orange with a banana and two greengages on a plate eaten with a knife and fork. Two of each of these per day can be added to larger items: plums/greengages/ apricots/figs/ prunes. Half a grapefruit, apple, melon, banana or pear can all be staple, varied larger fruits but no more than three items should be eaten per breakfast. Treat breakfasts are of course not to be denied and should be eaten a couple of times a week!

Carbohydrates for lunch around midday, salads, chicken or egg sandwiches not tuna/salmon, hot soups and stews, small desserts, plenty of pre-meal water, lots of vegetables should keep you going, elevate the immune system and control Candida.

Vegetables, like fruits, need rotation and variety. Wind producers like beans, broccoli, sprouts, cauliflower, swedes, parsnips, turnips, beetroot, cabbage, spinach, peas and onions are full of vitamins and minerals and so we need them, but only in moderation. They should be washed and peeled to remove surface moulds as well as crop spray residue. Buy organics wherever possible or grow your own in uncontaminated soil on an allotment or the back garden.

Carrots, watercress, lettuce, celery, and other raw leaves which, well washed in safe water, not Brita which has the highest metal content of all water filter systems, but an under-sink cartridge product like the Franke triflow system from John Lewis stores, are purer. Osmosis water filter systems or distilled water are far safer and better at removing metals.

Most desserts cause problems for Candida sensitive people, especially chocolate pies, mousses, gateaux, ice creams etc. Floury, sugary desserts like pies, crumbles, tarts and others slow peristalsis and encourage bacteria and yeasts to reproduce in greater numbers. Avoid flour-based desserts more than once a week. It goes without saying that ice-cream is a real no-no, unless you make other dietary preparations and restrictions and your current levels of Candida control are very high.

Beware any Candida cookbooks. It is easy enough not to cook with yeast or yeasty foods, but be sure to scrutinise any recipe ingredients for other known trouble-makers. Anti-Candida recipes may be alright for occasional reference but as a daily effort it is inevitable that you will lose interest and revert to bad habits. Anti-Candida books that concentrate only on diet are short-sighted and misleading. It is not merely a matter of food and drink but of background causes determining whether an already loaded immune system can withstand the effects of a cheese sandwich or glass of wine without causing a candida upsurge.

Before any meal drink water, but avoid drinking during the meal, just have an occasional sip if necessary. Since we need lots of gastric juice to deal with food entering the acid stomach, we don't want to dilute it with gulps of liquid. Digestion will be impaired, acidity will struggle to cope and food chunks, instead of sludge, will take longer to liquify later. Chew well before swallowing and ease pressure on stomach and intestinal processes.

All sweet drinks, carbonated waters, beers, lagers, ales, wines, spirits, liqueurs are death to the Candida sufferer. If an occasional 'treat' can be kept solely as a treat and not be allowed back into daily life as a habit, then go ahead; if not, regard it as OUT forever. If you are prepared to deal with the possible results of upsurge, then take the risk and deal with any miserable outcome. Apart from immediate glucose intake and natural digestive production of glucose, there's the matter of the crop spray chemicals and moulds on hops and grapes. Carbonated waters and drinks have added soda to make bubbles! This is alkaline, thrush loves it.

I like to give myself the power of control and balance. I am usually terribly careful, but I can be tempted if, for instance, there is a delicious wine on the table. Then it's a split-second decision to drink or not to drink. This will involve a computation of how good, or not, I have recently been in my avoidance and restrictions or whether the social occasion merits any possible consequence.

My own typical work day food may be:

Breakfast
Water on waking, then porridge cooked in semi-skimmed milk and a light covering of brown sugar. Afterwards, I may have a herbal tea or just hot, boiled water. In summer, I have three pieces of fruit.

Mid-morning
Another herbal tea or hot water, or decaffeinated coffee.

Lunch
A glass of water before, then leftovers from dinner the previous night, fried vegetables with a fried egg, soup, salad, meat, vegetables, whatever.

Mid-afternoon
More drink and a slice of hot, buttered toast.

Dinner (about 6.30-7.00 p.m., no later)
Meat and salad with potato mayonnaise, grated carrots sprinkled with chopped almonds and a few raisins, half a tomato, any amount of lettuce. This may be followed by a piece of cake or a small portion of any ordinary dessert like apple pie. I don't drink anything during the meal but only before and slightly after.

At weekends, depending upon any entertaining, there may be pasta, chops, salads, hot vegetables, a cooked breakfast, muesli, croissants, tea-cakes, and pretty much a normal array of foodstuffs. I can limit my own portions of suspect items and can pull myself right back out of a threatening Candidal upsurge. Overall, I could say that I do well enough for my background predisposition. I would love to have a sherry every evening, a glass of cider or wine most nights and include all the banned foods. I can't, though, if I want to live the rest of my life unhindered by my old, familiar enemy. It is comforting to realise how good my skills at controlling Candida are, and even more comforting not to have some other life-wrecking problem or injury which could restrict my life far more than Candida.

    I do not eat fish at all because it contains the highest amount of mercury of all foodstuffs, next are mushrooms. Even after amalgam removal I am warned not eat fish at all because scientists at the cutting edge of mercury recovery suggest that Alzheimers could be triggered. Fishing licenses in the States all carry warnings about not eating more than a pound of caught salmon because of the danger of mercury poisoning. Autopsied brains of Alzheimer victims show more mercury than aluminium and aluminium has been shown not to cause the amyloid plaques found in Alzheimer brains, only mercury has been shown to cause plaques.

If you feel odd any time within 24 hours of eating fish perhaps with decreased memory, lethargy, joint stiffness, digestive upset, stuffy nose or anything else, it may be the fish you ate. Worst are tuna, salmon, cod, most large fish, lobsters, mussels, crab and crustacea. Mercury bubbles up naturally from the sea floor. Crustacea and flat fish on the sea floor absorb much mercury, larger fish eat them and ingest this mercury plus sea-borne mercury. It is an accumulative effect. We eat all this and can get sick. If you drop just one mercury filling into a ten acre lake all fish and water becomes mercury contaminated.

At the end of this self-help chapter, I hope you realise how much control within daily living you have. As with cystitis, Candida can be very effectively reduced or eliminated. It is not just by diet; it is also by finding another or many lifestyle reasons for frequent upsurges or continual elevations of Candida. Examine everything, from swimming to soaps, from sex to supplements and from sadness to sweat. Get the mercury fillings out safely with proper removal protections and reduce immune system distress. Insist on white composite fillings, not glass ionomers. Look for anti-mercury books in bookshops or read my website and the PAMA Compilation at www.angela.kilmartin.dial.pipex.com

Stop modern Candida by prevention.

11 Common questions asked about Candida

I get fed up with asking my doctor to take vaginal swabs. Is there anywhere else that I could go?

Yes, Special Clinics or Sexual Health Clinics or Genito-Urinary Clinics. Phone the nearest hospital and ask for the telephone number of their clinic, whatever they call it, and find out whether an appointment is necessary or whether, in emergencies, it offers a walk-in facility. The staff are usually absolutely wonderful, and the facilities are far better than those found in general practice. I send all age groups and both sexes to them, and I use my own whenever I need to. By law they must see you if you say that you think you have a vaginal/penile discharge.

What is the link between myalgic encephalomyelitis (ME) and Candida?

Any severe illness strains the immune system, and ME is just such a one. Taking large doses of magnesium, plenty of zinc and folic acid are necessary for a long while. Insomnia and sleep-pattern disturbance must be controlled by sleeping aids such as herbal medicines or even occasional sleeping pills. Loss of sleep depletes the immune response. Eat well at breakfast and lunch, eat whenever you need to but go easy on a heavy supper. Take plenty of Bee Propolis and start EPD injections. Carry out the anti-Candida recommendations of this book and anything else relevant to keeping it at bay. Many ME and MS patients are suffering from mercury poisoning. With safe dental amalgam removal many regain their life.

What are safe amalgam removal procedures?

It is vital when seriously ill that safe removal of mercury fillings is practiced. A strong course of multi-minerals and vitamins should have been taken for ten days before treatment. Minimally, patient protection involves taking charcoal upon arrival at the dentist's, being totally covered up, having wet gauze over eyes and nose, wearing a comfortable oxygen mask. The dentist should have a well-ventilated room, isolate the tooth with a rubber dam, use high speed drill and close suction. The dentist and nurse must be gowned and masked because of mercury vapour and particulate spewing up at them. Dental staff still has the highest rates of professional suicide, foetal abnormality, miscarriage and infertility. Refuse any other method of removal.

Is there a recommended salad dressing for Candida-prone people?
Yes. Make the main ingredient a yoghurt and then add salt, pepper, some drops of lemon juice to taste and maybe a spoonful of mayonnaise. Other than vinegars of any kind, the basic recipe can be varied with mustards of all sorts, herbs, chives, garlic and so on. Just experiment. If salads are eaten daily, mayonnaise might be better than lemon juice.

Should fruit pieces be peeled or not?
All fruit these days should be peeled because of the use of insecticides. These contain cocktails of chemicals that impact upon sensitive immune systems and digestion. Additionally, fruit itself attracts aerial moulds and fungi. Remember to eat fruit sparingly because of the sugar content and fermentation during digestion. Tinned fruits are preserved in sugar syrups and the tin can leaks metals so avoid all tinned items.

My entire wardrobe consists of trousers or jeans. Must I really stop wearing them?
Yes, if you want to stop vaginal thrush and avoid other Candida upsurges. These garments may very well be the cause of your vulval Candida, if that's the trouble. If your job demands wearing trousers, then switch to divided skirts or culottes. These can be very sexy if well cut! Candida hates cooling air so keep cool down below!

How can I avoid sexual transference of Candida?
It's back to the condom, if you are sure that intercourse is responsible. It's always hard to prove this, unless a specific upsurge can be related to an event. Perhaps antibiotics were taken for something, or perhaps swimming recently has caused the upsurge. And I have mentioned the 'beer belly' problem before!

What is the commonest form of diet-related thrush?
Without a doubt, it is cheese on or in sandwiches, rolls, salads or toast. After that come chocolate, canned or bottled drinks and alcohol of all sorts. Sugar, mushrooms, vinegars, great chunks of fresh bread, yeast extract, canned fruits, too much fresh fruit and all the many foodstuffs which pander to the modern sweet

tooth. Stop, restrict, avoid, reduce, rotate are the buzz words.

My doctor is hopeless and refuses to discuss Candida with me. Who else can I turn to?

It may be necessary to see another doctor in the practice if it is not a sole practice, but you can also ask to change practices nowdays without a great fuss. If you live in a remote area, books become quite vital. Have your own copies, so that they are there for reference when required. Try putting an advert in a local paper for other sufferers and see whether it might be worth starting a self-help group to help everyone keep on the right path.

What should I do if I really have to take antibiotics?

Take the shortest course possible for the illness, in agreement with the doctor, and don't cut this down, since the infection may recur, and need more antibiotics. *Always* take an oral anti-fungal treatment as well, continuing for several days after the antibiotics have finished. Step up every rule in the book that might prevent a real upsurge occurring about ten days after the first day of the antibiotics. Remember that antibiotic action continues for at least one week, possibly five, depending upon the strength and duration of the course.

Should I come off the contraceptive pill?

If the Candida can be related to the start of taking the contraceptive pill, then yes, two and two make four! However, try another kind and/or step up all anti-Candida rules, since it may be these that are letting you down. If the Candida has arisen without a definite link to the Pill, then although it may be a part of the picture, it may not be the whole picture. Some other factor has entered and flipped the balance. Try and find this intruder first before abandoning a perfectly good contraceptive.

This sounds silly, but my child has bad athlete's foot and refuses to give up his trainers, which he wears all day. What can I do?

Let him suffer, refuse all creams, all lotions and visits to the doctor until it is just so bad that he has to give in. He has to stop wearing them and that's that. The longer he refuses to see sense and let air heal the fungus the longer his feet will need anti-fungal creams. Nothing else will help. Good shoe shops stock other, 'breathing' shoes. Bolster his courage and let him learn to admire these sorts of shoes, as well as telling his mates that the doctor has forbidden him to wear the trainers that are causing him to be ill.

Green vegetables cause me indigestion, to put it mildly! Obviously I need the minerals and vitamins from these sources, so what can I substitute, if anything?

First, try and eat less of them, but do so on alternate days. Before trying this, it may help to reduce Candida levels to a point where there is no bloating or wind. When you begin the new alternate-day diet, eat the windy vegetables at lunchtime so that they can be better digested and better monitored. If you feel happier with well-boiled greens, then boil them, otherwise carrots, lettuce, raw spinach and small amounts of raw greens of some sort may fit the bill. If not, then a daily supplement in tablet or capsule form should be taken to optimise body requirements.

I find the strict, anti-Candida diet that I was recently put on extremely hard to maintain over time. I have lost weight and feel weaker. What should I do?

Basically eat well and lots of it to restore your weight. Weight loss for Candida victims, unless you were very overweight, can only cause additional lethargy and weakness, which in turn helps Candida. These restriction diets can cause severe weight loss, depression, illness and are completely impractical. Allergy sufferers who also have Candida should really address the de-sensitisation programmes offered by EPD practitioners. Total food avoidance can sometimes lead to lessened tolerance of them once they are restored to the diet.

I have lived abroad and have had various illnesses such as dysentery, malaria and hepatitis. Would such bad health be responsible now for constant Candida?

It may well have depleted and damaged some of the immune defences, yes. Presumably, many drugs were taken to treat the conditions, which might have added to the damage as well. Liver function and sugar control may have been influenced long term, thereby enhancing nutrition for Candida growth. All the anti-Candida rules need to be solidly in place and continuous.

Which is better, Nystatin tablets or powders?

If the upsurge is simple and Candida does not reign in your body, then Nystatin tablets during and after a course of antibiotics should be sufficient. If it is a longer, anti-Candida therapy that you require just for dealing with intestinal Candida, then the powder form, also prescribable, is better. Probiotic therapy may be used instead or as an adjunct to the Nystatin.

I seem to get Candida when I sit my exams at university. What is causing this?

Probably several things. Sensible eating habits, sleep, rest and times to sit or stand are put aside as revision and study become feverish. Alcohol intake may be increased and chocolate snacks feature prominently. Obviously tiredness depletes the body's ability to throw off upsurges, and the week of exams finds people sitting for unnatural periods at a desk under pressure of time, as well as the seat and the jean seam!

What, would you say, are the extremes of Candida infestation?

Probably anything from a mild case of thrush in the mouth of a baby through to finding it as a contributory cause of death in the last days of a severely ill or starved person. There are a million stops in between these, and a million different lifestyle causes for upsurges.

My aunt was put on tranquilisers in the 1960s and has been tired ever since. Is there any chance that this could be Candida and if so, how can I help her?

If your aunt has been on these drugs permanently, then her system will have become used to them. If she wishes to come off them, it will be a long, hard, road to travel. Look for books on this subject. Every process in the body would have been slowed and altered in some way. This means that natural healthy resistance to Candidal upsurge has been put at risk, and, as my chapter on medicines shows, such drugs can promote fungal infections.

Will I always be prone to Candida?

Not necessarily. It depends upon all the background factors being present or absent; it depends upon the amount of mercury or other dental metals like chrome cobalt from dentures leaking into your body; it depends upon any medications needed for any illnesses; it depends upon levels of hormones; it depends upon workloads and tiredness; it depends upon clothing, diet, liquids and all the other factors shown in this book. It depends primarily on how much control and care you exert on your own body to keep it as fresh and well as possible.

Do you advise many people in counselling to move house, change jobs or slow down?

Some certainly need to re-think their entire life, but most do not, since Candida can often be stopped by one or two small changes. Systemic Candida is another matter and absolutely everything contributing to it has to be re-thought. If every part of the body is involved and life quality threatened, then changing job, house or anything else just has to be considered.

Why do so many vaginal swabs return a negative result?

This may happen if you are not at the peak of the problem, if a pessary was used that week, if you washed out the discharge before going for the swab, if the sample was kept in the fridge because the microbiology department was closed, if the sample was carelessly stored, if it is not Candida at all but another white vaginal discharge called non-infective leucorrhoea which, in quantity, can also itch and inflame, if you have taken any oral anti-fungal treatment recently.

Would diabetics benefit from self-help?

Certainly, but their problem is balancing sugar levels. The presiding doctor or specialist should be involved with all self-help dietary decisions, contributing ideas in keeping with the individual's needs. This book has lots of ideas that might be helpful but discussion may be needed.

In counselling, dozens of questions and answers flow back and forth between practitioner and patient. These have been just a small selection of more general topics about Candida.

Are there any new medications available from the doctor?

For ten years a new conventional, prescribable medication for fungal infections has been in the pipeline. It is called "Immune 26" and is basically a product made from egg yolk. Information can be found from www.legacyforlife.com . However, although rigorously tested one never knows quite what effects will be discovered twenty years down the line. The self help in this book is very safe and managed by the patient not by prescription from a doctor, as such it is always the first and best option.

CHAPTER 12

12 Summary

This book has sought to fill a gap. Since it is neither a short patient's guide nor a large medical textbook but a mixture of both, it is to be hoped that doctors will come to regard it as an easy-to-read but medically authoritative work. Doctors Truss, Crook and Chaitow have done wonders in turning the spotlight publicly onto Candida through their researches and practices in America. They have moved practical treatments, immune system knowledge and modern causes of candidosis/monilia/fungal/yeast infections and thrush right out into the public arena. Many books are now available but this one deals with background causes and determines how to deal effectively with them in order to limit fungal upsurges. Certainly the very considerable research which I have undertaken both as sufferer and counsellor, has proved extraordinarily exciting and stimulating.

I don't begin to pretend that I could quote chapter and verse on body systems, and it is not essential for patients to understand all the minutiae of inter-dependent actions. I have tried, though, to lead the reader step-by-step from various starting points. It has perhaps had something of a maypole feel about it - the pole for Candida and several coloured ribbons which, when woven correctly, should all end neatly at the bottom, forming a completed process with a decrease in symptoms. I hope that all, or a great many, useful ideas and known facts have been brought out, aired and offered as solutions in part, in total or in conjunction with someone's own personal situation.

It has been a great relief to see clearly and to have research proof from several sources that many people can become Candida sufferers. This may be determined by body system malfunctions; enzyme malfunctions; endocrine malfunctions; immune system damage; mercury poisoning from teeth fillings; digestive system damage and a weakened general health in all ages of sufferers. These sorts of conditions would have been equally preponderant throughout the centuries, although, before microscopes, it would have been impossible to prove. Even so, significant writers on health and medicine down through the ages have noted much evidence in the mouth, the vagina, the gut and the anus of 'irritation, white flux, curds, plaques, spots, wind, bloated belly, itchy anus' and the rest of it. I no longer believe that Candida is as modern an illness as I had previously thought.

Modern additions to daily living, such as antibiotics, steroids, contraceptives, additives, sugars, allergies, sleeping pills, tranquilisers and anaesthetics, are certainly new to the world's population. It is the over-use and abuse of many of them that our metabolism simply cannot tolerate, and beers, breads, fruits, wines and poor foodstuffs were just as capable of causing fungal overloads in years gone by.

I have just taken a phone call, as I write, from a thirteen-year-old patient of mine who visited me a month ago with her distraught mother. The girl has just achieved her first free week from Candida and urethral twinges since my plans for a lifestyle reappraisal were recommended. This young girl has been so uncomfortable and miserable for two years that she has had to study at home and lose the companionship of her school friends. In counselling, she was taught the bottle-washing, stopped from taking the normal, lengthy baths which teenagers take, and had her high sugar and chocolate snacks removed. After countless visits to doctors, the logical, simple lifestyle revisions have once again proved their worth. She and her mother are very grateful.

There are no conventional specialists in Candida Albicans. We, the patients, would like this situation to change. There are specialists in allergies and private, expensive doctors dealing with Candida de-sensitisation. Together with lifestyle changes, de-sensitisation may have a place for many victims. But amalgam removal has for me been the best treatment for constant Candida. Rigid diets are daunting, unrealistic and weakening. Many sufferers feel likewise.

However, the ideas and treatments herein are because I want to stress *CHOICE*. Each sufferer has a unique order to their daily life and must therefore choose treatments appropriately.

The telephone has rung again. This time a patient whose general practitioner has firmly refused to acknowledge the existence or possibility of Candida in the bladder! When such a situation arises, I would hope this book will be used as evidence, and if more is required, then suggest that the doctor in question reads the section on bladder Candida in Professor Odds' book, *Candida and Candidosis*. Many research papers have long since proved this aspect.

I would also like to thank the various nutritional supplement and therapy manufacturers for those products which safeguard intestinal balance. These are enormously helpful therapies which, by their very presence, comfort Candida sufferers who would otherwise be totally at the mercy of ignorant doctors.

Finally, the time has come to acknowledge Candida Albicans, its sub-strains and all other fungi and yeasts, as being equal in importance to bacterial infections. Life now is such that we must take Candida very seriously - it certainly costs enough in terms of suffering and medications. Neither doctors nor patients can afford to continue in the current air of ignorance.

APPENDIX - EPD PRACTITIONERS

Dr Damien Downing
Galtres House
Lysander Close
York Y03 8XB
Tel: 01904 691591 Appts
Fax:01904 690588
Also at Biolab in London, Windsor in Berkshire, Harlow Mill in Hertfordshire

Dr S.Z. Haider and others at
Royal London Homeopathic Hospital
Great Ormond Street
London WC1N 3HR
Tel: 0207 837 8833
This clinic is not private, but all others are.

Dr L M. McEwen and Dr Helen C. McEwen
Weir View
Wargrave Road,
Henley on Thames
RG9 1HX
01491 576314

Please write to Dr. Mc Ewen for updated lists of all other national and international practitioners.

GLOSSARY

aerobic - descriptive term for bacteria that need oxygen to grow.

anaerobic - descriptive term for bacteria that do not need oxygen to grow.

bacillus - rod-shaped bacteria derived from plant life. B cell cell which secretes antibodies to help fight infection.

cell - a tiny speck of protein held in shape by a membranous coating.

chyme - food particles now turned into a brown liquid in small intestine.

disaccharide - sugar formed from two hexoses, such as glucose, fructose or galactose.

DNA - Deoxyribo Nucleic Acid; the genetic blueprint of all life.

enzyme - a chemical substance formed within the body, activating chemical or bacterial changes, but not needing to change in itself.

fermentation - a process whereby sugar is converted into energy by bacteria and yeasts as carbon dioxide, gas and alcohol.

hexose - a group of sugars formed from a monosaccharide.

immunity - the power held by the immune system enabling bacterial, viral and fungal balance through good health.

lysozyme - an enzyme found in body secretion which dissolves bacteria.

micro-organism - any minute, microscopic plant or animal.

monosaccharide - one simple sugar.

OTC - over the counter, no prescription required.

parasite - a plant or animal needing a host upon which to live.

pH - potential of hydrogen; the acid to alkaline measurement (pH 1 is very acid, pHl4 very alkaline; blood pH is 7.4, urine 6.4 approximately).

proteins - compounds needed by all living plants and animals to sustain healthy tissues and fluids.

putrefaction - decomposition of plant or animal life by micro-organisms.

rhinitis - inflammation of the nasal mucus membrane.

T cell - a cell derived from the thymus gland in the neck.

toxin a - poisonous substance produced by bacterial action.

thrush - another name for Candida.

REFERENCES

Balding, Peter, *The Battle against Bacteria*, Cambridge, Cambridge University Press, 1965

Billings, Frank, *Modern Clinical Medicine*, New York, D. Appleton & Co., 1910

Blanchard, C.E., *The Romance of Proctology*, Ohio, Medical Success Press, 1938

Casarett & Doull, *Toxicology. the basic science of poisons*, McGraw Hill 5th ed., 1996

Chaitow, Leon and Trenev, Natasha, *Probiotics*, London, Thorsons, 1990

Cleave, Captain T.L., *The Saccharine Disease*, Bristol, John Wright & Sons Ltd, 1974

Dwyer, Professor John, *The Body at War*, London, J.M. Dent, 1993

Eberson, Frederick, *Microbes Militant: A Challenge to Man*, New York, The Ronald Press Company, 1948

Gabriel, William, *The Principles and Practice of Rectal Surgery*, London, H.K. Lewis & Co. Ltd, 1948

Huggins, Dr Hal DDS, MS, *It's All in Your Head*, New York, Avery Publishing Group, 1993

Last, Walter, *Heal Yourself*. Australia, Viking O'Neill, 1991 Norbury, L.E., *Proctology throughout the Ages (the Bradshaw Lecture of 1948)*, The Royal College of Surgeons

Odds, F.C. PhD, MRC, *Candida and Candidosis*, London, Balliere Tindall, 1988

Penn, R.G. MG, *Pharmacology*, London, Balliere Tindall, 3rd ed., 1980

Playfair, J.H.L., *Immunology at a GLance*, Oxford, Blackwell Scientific Publications, 5th ed., 1992

Ricci, James MD, *One Hundred Years of Gynecology*, Philadelphia, Blakiston, 1945

Robertson, J.D. MD, CP, *Gastric Acidity*, London, John Murray for Middlesex Hospital Press, 1931

Sanford, Paul, *Digestive System Physiology*, London, Edward Arnold, 1992

Scheibner Dr Viera, Ph.D. *Vaccinations*. Pub: Scheibner NSW, Australia 1993

Smith, Dr Mike, *Handbook of Prescription Medicines*, London, Lyle Cathie, 1994

Stewart-McKay, WJ. *History of Ancient Gynaecology*, London, Balliere, Tindall & Cox, 1901

Trimmer, Dr Eric, *The Magic of Magnesium*, London, Thorsons, 1987

Truelove and Reynell, *Diseases of the Digestive System*, Oxford, Blackwell Scientific Publishers, 1903

Underwood, Michael, *Treatise on the Diseases of Children*, London, Matthews, 1784

Wainwright, Milton, *Miracle Cure*, Cambridge, Mass., Blackwell Ltd, 1990

Wingate, Peter, *Medical Encyclopaedia*, London, Penguin Books, 1972

INDEX